W9-CMF-541

*Praise for*

# NICOLE HUNN

"Even when she's telling you something you think you already know—like grow your own vegetables—Hunn adds an extra bit of information that takes the wisdom to another level."

—Epicurious.com

"Hunn has not only bestowed her readers with a complete cookbook . . . but she shows us how to save money, and time, on our meals . . . It's well worth a bite."

—*San Francisco Book Review*

"No childhood favorites are off-limits with *Gluten-Free Classic Snacks* by author/blogger Nicole Hunn of *Gluten-Free on a Shoestring*. Expect recipe riffs on Twinkies, Thin Mints, Nutter Butters, Pop-Tarts, and more in her ode to edible Americana."

—*GFF Magazine*

"Nicole Hunn serves up all the recipes and information found in her cookbook in the friendly and inviting manor that has helped make her blog popular."

—National Foundation for Celiac Awareness

"Hunn is clever and optimistic. As you flip through the pages, it's hard to avoid not feeling better about your gluten-free life. Plus, the recipes will inspire you to go into the kitchen with renewed energy and hope for the future. It's well worth spending money to purchase *Gluten-Free on a Shoestring*. It will pay dividends in the future."

—*Gluten-Free Living*

"I highly recommend [*Gluten-Free on a Shoestring Quick & Easy*]. The recipes are accessible and especially geared for people with busy lifestyles."

—*Tucson Citizen*

"With plenty of wisdom and easy instructions, *Gluten-Free on a Shoestring* is a must for any gluten-intolerant, health-conscious cook."

—*Midwest Book Review*

"Hunn successfully tackles a chief complaint voiced by special-diet newbies: sticker shock. Her practical tips for shopping and cooking to save time and money are a gift to all of us who are paying too much for too little."

—*Living Without*

"The money you spend on the book will be saved by following Hunn's great tips."

—*TheSavvyCeliac.com*

"Compiles [Hunn's] best recipes and helpful hints on cutting costs, all in best friend blogger-style. Her tips to economizing are good reminders and handy for the working parent."

—*Marin Independent Journal*

"Opens up a whole new world for people with this particular diet restriction and does so with a writing style that is both assured and accessible. Those of us who don't have a medical diagnosis requiring diet changes can benefit from the book, as well . . . Hunn's book gives everyone a map toward healthier eating without giving up those delicious foods we love."

—*Curled Up With a Good Book*

"From locating best values to meal planning and stocking a gluten-free pantry, this provides a range of foods from 'scratch' that can fit any budget. Highly recommended!"

—*Midwest Book Review*

"This book is written for real people, facing real economic issues, that can't afford to dedicate a whole paycheck to groceries. It is a great resource for preparing whole foods at home and not spending all weekends and evenings in the kitchen."

—*Portland Book Review*

# GLUTEN-FREE
## ON A
*Shoestring*
*Second Edition*

*Also by*
NICOLE HUNN

*Gluten-Free Small Bites*

*Gluten-Free Classic Snacks*

*Gluten-Free on a Shoestring Bakes Bread*

*Gluten-Free on a Shoestring Quick & Easy*

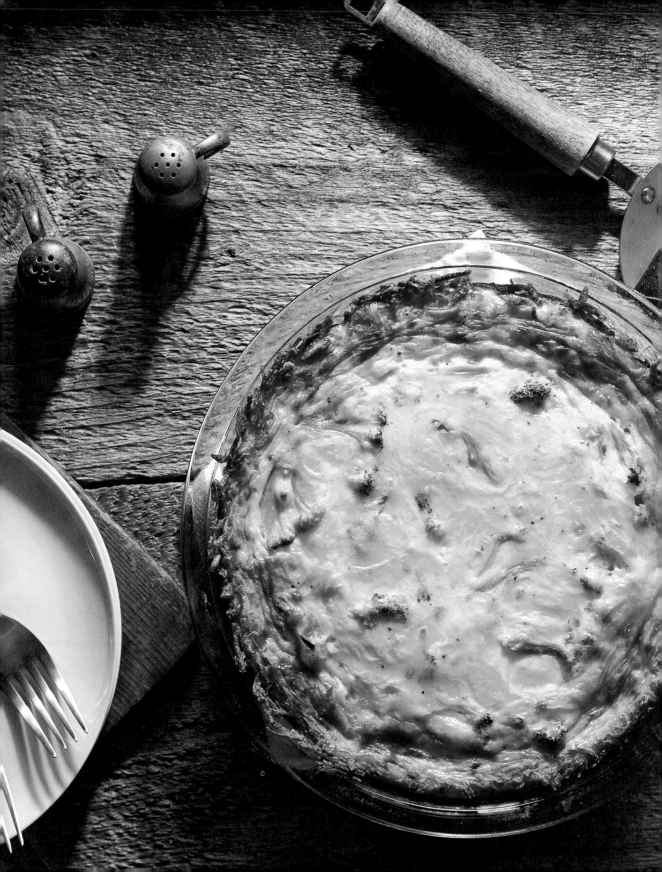

# GLUTEN-FREE

## ON A

# Shoestring

### ~Second Edition~

## 125 EASY RECIPES FOR
## EATING WELL ON THE CHEAP

## Nicole Hunn

Da Capo

LIFE
LONG

Many of the designations used by manufacturers and
sellers to distinguish their products are claimed as
trademarks. Where those designations appear in this book
and Da Capo Press was aware of a trademark claim, the
designations have been printed in initial capital letters.

Copyright © 2017 by Nicole Hunn

Hachette Book Group supports the right to free
expression and the value of copyright. The purpose of
copyright is to encourage writers and artists to produce
the creative works that enrich our culture.

The scanning, uploading, and distribution of this book
without permission is a theft of the author's intellectual
property. If you would like permission to use material from
the book (other than for review purposes), please contact
permissions@hbgusa.com. Thank you for your support of
the author's rights.

Da Capo Press
Hachette Book Group
1290 Avenue of the Americas, New York, NY 10104
www.dacapopress.com
@DaCapoPress

Printed in the United States of America

Originally published in paperback and ebook by
Da Capo Press in February 2011.

Second Edition: October 2017

Published by Da Capo Press an imprint of
Perseus Books, LLC, a subsidiary of
Hachette Book Group, Inc.

The Hachette Speakers Bureau provides a wide
range of authors for speaking events. To find out
more, go to www.hachettespeakersbureau.com or
call (866) 376-6591.

The publisher is not responsible for websites
(or their content) that are not owned by the publisher.

Photographs by Jean Schwarzwalder
Food styling by Derek Laughren.
Book design by Shubhani Sarkar, sarkardesignstudio.com

Library of Congress Cataloging-in-Publication Data
has been applied for.

ISBNs: 978-0-7382-1986-8 (paperback);
978-0-7382-1987-5 (ebook)

LSC-C

10  9  8  7  6  5  4  3  2  1

FOR MY HUSBAND,
*Brian*

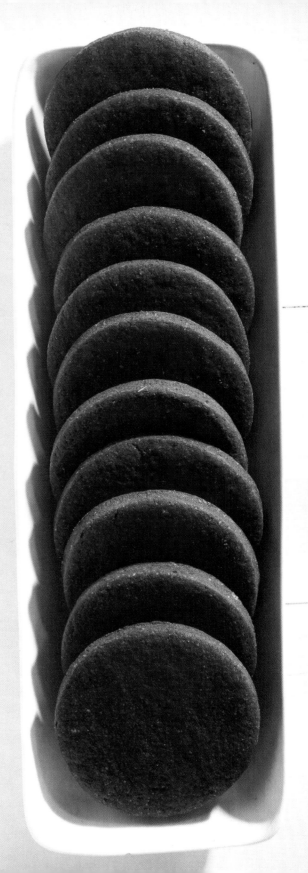

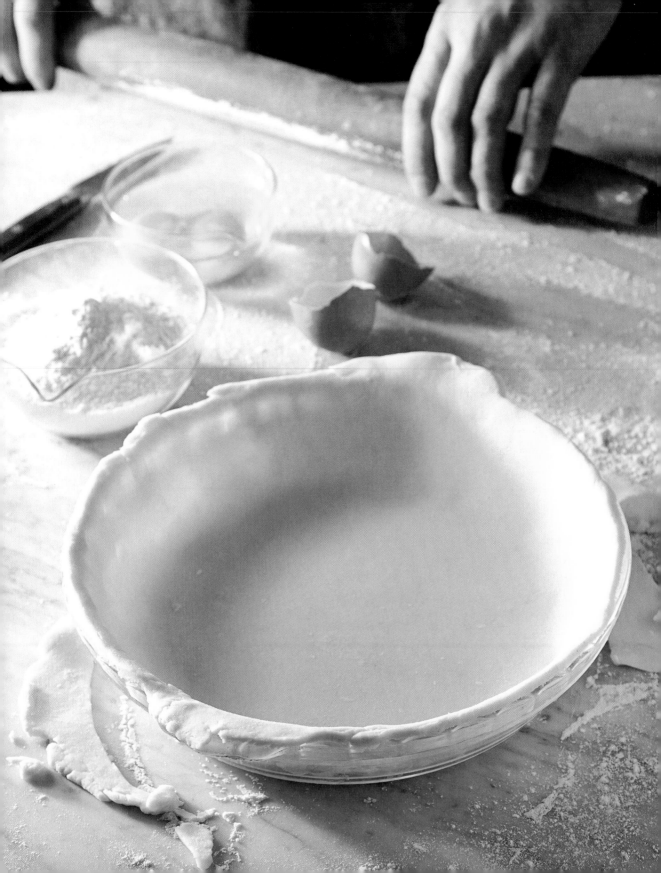

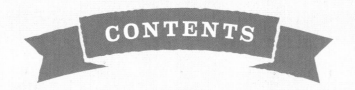

# CONTENTS

PREFACE TO THE SECOND EDITION   xv

INTRODUCTION   xvii

### SHOESTRING STRATEGIES: SAVING AT THE STORE AND IN YOUR KITCHEN

Tip #1: Use Coupons                                    2

Tip #2: Practice Once-a-Week Cooking                   4

Tip #3: Practice One-a-Month Cooking                   4

Tip #4: Piggyback Your Meals                           5

Tip #5: Stretch Your Food                              6

Tip #6: Be Smart About
How You Store Your Food                                7

Tip #7: If It's on Sale, Buy in Bulk                   7

Tip #8: Grow a Vegetable Garden                        7

Tip #9: Buy Frozen Veggies                             8

### WHAT TO BUY AND FROM WHERE

The Well-Stocked, Gluten-Free,
Shoestring-Friendly Pantry                            10

Pantry Staples                                        11

To Market, to Market:
What to Buy Weekly at the Grocery                     12

Ordering Online                                       14

The Best Gluten-Free Values
and the Best Places to Find Them                      16

Essential Kitchen Equipment                           16

If You're Dairy-Free, Too                             18

Gluten-Free Flour Blends                              19

### KITCHEN CONFIDENCE: BASIC RECIPES THAT SERVE AS THE FOUNDATION FOR MANY OTHERS

#### Meal Ingredients                                 25

Chicken Stock                                         26

Scratch Black Beans                                   28

#### Doughs and Crusts                                29

Sweet Pastry Crust                                    31

Savory Pastry Crust                                   32

Savory Olive Oil Crust                                33

Fresh Pasta Dough                                     35

Pizza Dough                                           36

Wonton Wrappers                                       38

Pâte à Choux                                          40

Gougères (Cheese Puffs)                               43

Profiteroles (Cream Puffs)                            43

#### Sauces and Soups                                 44

Easy Enchilada Sauce                                  45

Chinese-Style Hot Sauce                               46

Sweet and Sour Sauce                                  46

Hoisin Sauce                                          47

Barbecue Sauce                                        47

Easy Homemade Tomato Sauce                            48

Cream of Mushroom Soup                                49

Cream of Chicken Soup                                 50

Cream of Potato Soup                                  51

Dips and Snacks 52

Spinach Dip 53

Traditional Hummus 54

Homemade Jell-O-Style Gelatin 55

Cheese Crackers 57

## BREAKFAST AND BRUNCH, JUST AS YOU REMEMBER THEM

Tortilla Española 60

Oven Hash Brown Quiche 63

Ricotta Pancakes 64

Buttermilk Pancakes 67

Banana Pancake Muffins 68

Soft and Fluffy Waffles 70

Easy Oatmeal Breakfast Cookies 71

Apple-Cinnamon Toaster Pastries 72

Homemade Crunchy Granola 75

Plain Bagels 76

Cinnamon Rolls 78

Berry Scones 81

Blueberry Muffins 82

Banana Muffins 85

Coffee Cake 86

Bread Pudding 88

Cheese Blintzes 89

Biscuits and Sausage Gravy 91

## THE GREATEST THING SINCE . . . BREAD, GLORIOUS BREAD

Old-Fashioned Cornbread 97

Cornmeal Flatbread 98

Dinner Rolls 99

Drop Biscuits 103

Buttermilk Biscuits 104

Sweet Potato Biscuits 107

White Sandwich Bread 109

English Muffin Bread 113

Brioche Bread 114

Irish Soda Bread 116

Soft Pretzels 119

Flour Tortillas 121

Popovers 125

Crêpes 126

## EAT YOUR VEGETABLES: MEATLESS MEALS AND SIDES

Corn and Zucchini Fritters 130

Sweet and Sour Beets 132

Glazed Carrots 133

Baked Eggplant Parmesan 135

Potato Gnocchi 137

Ricotta Gnocchi 139

Spinach and Cheese Ravioli 142

Lentil Sloppy Joes 145

Spinach Pie 146

Arepas 149

Crispy Asian-Style Tofu 150

Cornmeal Spoonbread 153

Tomato Polenta 154

Polenta Pizza 157

Zucchini Pizza 158

Noodle Kugel 159

Tomato Soup 160

Cheddar Broccoli Soup 161

## COMFORTING DINNERS: JUST LIKE MOM USED TO MAKE

Macaroni and Cheese   165

Apple-Leek-Sausage Cornbread Stuffing Dinner   166

Meatlove   168

Lo Mein   171

Szechuan Meatballs   172

Beef Potstickers   175

Sweet and Sour Chicken   176

Lemon Chicken, Chinese-Style   179

Asian Pork Loin   180

Chicken Potpie   181

Shepherd's Pie   185

Beef Potpie   186

Chicken en Croute   187

Chicken and Dumplings Soup   188

Matzoh Ball Soup   190

Tortilla Soup   191

Pot Roast   192

Chicken Enchiladas   193

Zucchini-Stuffed Chicken Parmesan Bundles   194

## ROOM FOR DESSERT: CAKES, COOKIES, AND PIES

Thick and Chewy Chocolate Chip Cookies   199

Crispy Gingerbread Men Cookies   200

Soft Ginger Cookies   202

Soft Frosted Sugar Cookies   203

Drop Sugar Cookies   207

Crispy Chocolate Wafer Cookies   208

Ladyfingers   211

Chocolate Chip Biscotti   212

Black and White Cookies   214

Butter Cookies   217

Cookie Breakup   219

Chocolate Sandwich Cookies   220

Chewy Sugar Cookies   221

Graham Crackers   222

Lemon Cupcakes   224

Chocolate Chip Blondie Cupcakes   226

Chocolate Chip Brownies   227

Flourless Brownies   229

No-Bake Cheesecake   230

Perfect Yellow Cake   232

Devil's Food Cake   235

Pound Cake   236

Perfect Chocolate Birthday Cake   239

Apple Cake   240

Pumpkin Bread   243

Pumpkin Chocolate Chip Squares   244

Pumpkin Pie with Ginger Cookie Crust   245

Banana Cream Pie with Graham Cracker Crust   247

Classic Apple Pie   249

Apple Crisp   253

Cheesecake with Butter Cookie Crust   254

Rice Pudding   257

Toppings   258

Basic White Frosting   259

Citrus Glaze   260

Sour Cream Chocolate Frosting   261

Royal Icing   262

METRIC CONVERSIONS   265

ACKNOWLEDGMENTS   267

INDEX   269

ABOUT THE AUTHOR   281

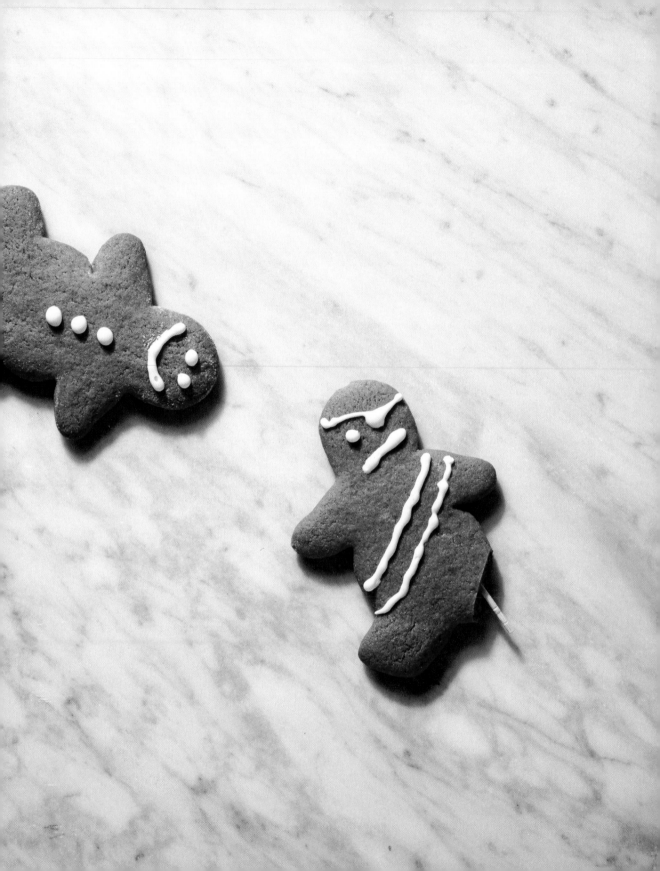

# PREFACE TO
# THE SECOND EDITION

OVER SIX YEARS HAVE PASSED SINCE THE PUBLICATION OF THE ORIGINAL EDITION OF THIS BOOK. IN the gluten-free world, so much has changed. We have more gluten-free products available to us than we had ever imagined possible. In many cases, they're even sharing shelf space with conventional foods. A gluten-free dream come true!

In my world, as much as things have changed, they've stayed the same as well. I've written four other cookbooks, but the blog is still strong, vibrant, and updated every week of every year. And I don't plan to stop.

In fact, I feel more obligated than ever to promise you, my reader, that I won't stop. I'll be here with you, every step of the way. As more gluten-free products become available to us, I will continue to be honest with you about what works and what doesn't. I will never be beholden to any one food or products company. I will continue to refuse to accept

free products, much to my husband and children's frustration. With every new book, every blog post and product I offer online, I ask you to trust me. And I must be worthy of that trust.

The original edition of this cookbook had no more than a few photos, and this edition has beautiful color photos throughout. But the difference between this edition and the first is much more than just visuals. Almost every corner of this cookbook has been edited and revised. We have taken pains, however, to strike that perfect balance between shiny new content that demonstrates what I have learned over the last six years and preservation of old content that merely needed a light touch or simple refinement to bring it up to date.

The most significant lesson in gluten-free cooking and baking that I have learned over the years has to be my understanding of gluten-free flours and blends. When I first wrote the original edition of this cookbook, just the idea of developing recipes around an "all-purpose gluten-free flour blend" was revolutionary. In fact, the book was criticized in some arenas for that aspect alone. Years later, I stand by that original decision. Baking with an all-purpose blend using well-crafted gluten-free recipes normalizes the whole process in a very important way. Especially when you first begin cooking and baking gluten-free, normalcy is the holy grail. However, not all all-purpose blends are created equal. I have a few brands that I recommend, and I have also worked hard to reverse engineer those blends to allow you to re-create them at home if you prefer not to, or are not able to, buy them ready-made.

Just as conventional all-purpose flour is good for all purposes but not ideal for every situation, so it is with all-purpose gluten-free flour blends. That's why the recipes in this book sometimes call for a very simple, basic three-ingredient gum-free gluten-free flour blend. It contains only white rice flour, potato starch, and tapioca starch, and it is a cooking essential—from creating a simple roux to thicken a sauce or gravy to making pancakes and certain cakes. In fact, I'm often told that the recipes that call for that blend are better tasting than their gluten counterparts, as the resulting dishes are as delicate as they are intended to be without gluten getting in the way of the texture.

All five of my gluten-free cookbooks are a labor of love, and I have an enormous sense of pride in each of them. I believe that they all will help you to live a better life, as food unites us every day. It should be a source of pleasure, not pain. It shouldn't separate us. This cookbook, the flagship book, is where we should all begin, and I promise you'll come back to this book most often. I know I do.

If you use these recipes, everyone in your family can enjoy the same meals, together. You'll be willing to host holidays, if that's your thing, and feel nothing but pride as you serve a gluten-free bounty. Just promise me you'll smile gently whenever you're asked for your recipe and say sweetly, "It's gluten-free, and I'm so glad you like it."

# INTRODUCTION

I'T'S NO SURPRISE THAT, NO MATTER HOW SPACIOUS THE HOUSE, GUESTS AND FAMILY MEMBERS ALWAYS HEAD for the kitchen like homing pigeons. That's where all the action is. And it's the cook who sets it in motion.

A good meal can leave a lasting impression; it can even make your day. And turning out a favorite dessert can make an otherwise ordinary meal into something memorable. All you need is some standard kitchen equipment, plus a few basic skills and recipes, and you're on your way. When you have the ability to cook, you can reward yourself and your family with homemade treats, tailoring every last detail to your own tastes. You can perk up your entire office with a simple batch of cookies or cupcakes. Or cater to a child's special birthday wish. Bake a loaf of bread, and you'll make any house smell like a home. As long as your pantry is well stocked with the basics, nothing is out of reach.

And none of that has to change when you're gluten-free.

First, a few basics. Gluten is the protein found primarily in wheat, barley, and rye. It is found in all conventional breads and pastas and is also frequently hidden in ingredients such as maltodextrin and dextrin, hydrolyzed vegetable protein, malt or malt flavoring, and modified food starch, all of which are often derived from gluten-containing ingredients. Increasingly, there are all sorts of people who eat a gluten-free diet in varying degrees, from the strictly gluten-free to the occasional gluten-free-food dabbler. Celiac disease is an autoimmune disease in which, in response to the ingestion of gluten, the body attacks itself by destroying villi, the finger-like projections in the lining of the small intestine that are responsible for the absorption of nutrients. The only treatment is to follow a completely gluten-free diet. Recent research indicates that celiac disease affects as many as 1 in 133

Americans, most of whom remain undiagnosed. Many others who do not have celiac disease choose to enjoy the benefits of a gluten-free diet as well, including those suffering from nonceliac gluten sensitivity, family members of celiacs, and those seeking various other general health benefits from the diet. Whether you're new to eating gluten-free and fear that the creative foodie part of your life is gone forever, or you've been gluten-free for a while and have resigned yourself to lowered expectations and expensive, store-bought gluten-free foods that leave you cold, help is on the way. Everything's going to be just fine.

All that being said, I must admit that it took me loads of trial and error to come to this state of gluten-free zen. When we discovered that my second child, Jonathan, had celiac disease, although I was thankful his condition didn't warrant a lifetime of expensive medications with possible side effects, I honestly didn't know the first thing about eating gluten-free. And I worried about how his dietary restriction would affect our entire family. So I started out by sticking with naturally gluten-free foods like vegetables, meats, and vegetarian proteins, like rice and beans. The only baking I was confident enough to try was with gluten-free mixes. At the time, I thought mixes were my only hope, and, frankly, I was grateful to have them. Without much experience with conventional mixes upon which to base my expectations, I just gave it a whirl. I don't want to tell tales out of school and spell out exactly which brands I tried, but suffice it to say that there was some weeping (me) and some queasiness (me, the kids, my husband). And there was also the whole unpleasantness

(my husband and me) about how much these experiments were costing us (a lot). I paid over $6 for a gluten-free cake mix, plus the cost of shipping and the cost of the ingredients that I had to add to the mix to make the cake. King Arthur Flour's gluten-free bread mix costs $7.99—just for the mix! But I took it on the chin and kept searching, assuming I just hadn't yet stumbled upon the right mix.

Time and time again, our thoughts turned wistfully to sandwiches. Initially we relied on packaged gluten-free bread. I remember this one particular bread that could be cured of that dense, gluten-free sponginess by toasting it. The only problem was that you had to eat it within moments. If you took the time, all five minutes of it, to actually make a simple turkey sandwich, the bread would spring back to its pretoasted, spongy form. I have to imagine that if a company set out intending to make bread with such unyielding resilience, they would have failed miserably.

I tried looking on the bright side: it looked good. This was one handsome slice of gluten-free bread. If you confined yourself to visual observation of a slice, it was a dead ringer for edible bread. And there appeared to be a whole community of gluten-free people online who thought this was the best gluten-free bread, upon whose endorsements we had based our mail order of a whole case of the stuff. But sadly, our best efforts to eat each slice straight out of the toaster proved impossible in the long run. And at about $7 a loaf, plus shipping, it was incompatible with our food budget.

All the while, our family's monthly expenses were growing by leaps and bounds, and we just weren't eating well. None of us felt quite right, but we didn't yet know where to turn.

Out of necessity I began to search, mostly online, for gluten-free recipes that I could make from scratch. At first, I experienced a renaissance of kitchen confidence, but it was short-lived. Many of the gluten-free recipes I found were full of ingredients that proved obscure and expensive, and the instructions were so complicated that, at times, I felt like I needed a degree in chemistry just to understand them. Did it really have to be so difficult? I started wondering if I couldn't do a better job on my own. After all, I was armed with necessity, the mother of invention.

Feeling otherwise trapped, I committed myself to trying to convert my repertoire of conventional recipes to gluten-free goodness. My first attempts at baking from scratch were, well, dismal failures. My cakes and bread tasted terrible, not to mention that they were these sad, weepy piles of dough. My cupcakes crumbled into tiny bits, along with my hopefulness (cue the violins). Finally, I started learning about all-purpose gluten-free flours that, with the addition of a binder called xanthan gum and some ratio modifications, could substitute cup for cup for conventional wheat flours. After two tries, I finally made a gluten-free carrot cake that looked pretty handsome—and tasted as good as it looked. I was back in business!

After a few more successes, and fewer outright failures, my experiments grew bolder. I began to hone my skills and refine my recipes, making them better and better. Finally, I realized that the sky was the limit—gluten-free or not—and that gluten-free cooking and baking doesn't have to be a daunting challenge when you focus on the right ingredients and have the right instruction.

### HOW TO SUCCEED IN GLUTEN-FREE WITHOUT REALLY TRYING

I started to realize that with a few simple tricks, I could reduce my family's grocery bills significantly, something that became more and more important as we felt the effects of the new economy. I went from spending, on average, $175 a week for groceries to spending less than $100 a week. And not only were we eating better, the food seemed more plentiful. Oddly enough, even though my husband and I were part of a celiac support group and more and more people we knew were avoiding gluten for one reason or another, the cost of living gluten-free was something that nobody seemed to be talking about—at least not at first. Only when I began to mention how we were saving all this money, always to a surprised and eager audience, did I begin to realize what an important, but under-the-radar, issue this had become. Since everyone wanted to know my secrets, I started a blog called Gluten-Free on a Shoestring. In short order, I began to enjoy gluten-free cooking and baking more and more. As both the blog and my collection of recipes grew, I began receiving scores of e-mails from readers, enthusiastic that saving money and living a gluten-free life full of flavor and possibilities were not mutually exclusive after all.

This book, as a natural extension of the website, represents the culmination of many years of hard work, experimentation, and perfection of recipes—created in response to the demands of both my family and my readers. You, too, can be in on the secret and learn to feed yourself, your family, and your guests fabulous gluten-free food—while still keeping an eye on the household budget. Think of how liberating it will be to satisfy your heart's desire in the kitchen, no worries about gluten or about the grocery bill. You'll soon feel freer to entertain, knowing that you can make a tasty, satisfying meal, complete with dessert, for everyone, even the most discriminating foodies.

The recipes in this book are not about making time-consuming, complicated, restaurant-quality food. They're about traditional staples, easy dinners, and comfort foods—the things that we all crave these days (the gluten-free among us even more). This approach will not only save you money but will allow you to feed your family consciously and deliberately—something that we all should do more often. And you'll reap the rewards when you hear your children literally sing while they eat their dinner, as do mine.

This cookbook is the flagship book of what has grown into the Shoestring cookbook series. It's the cookbook that started it all, and it proved a point. We want to eat well, to feed our families and friends well. We also want to prove something to the world: "good for gluten-free" simply isn't good enough. Our food must be good, period.

The first edition of this book was originally published in 2011. Four other cookbooks have followed, and the blog has grown by leaps and bounds. The mission is the same, and only the scope has broadened.

In that spirit, in addition to providing recipes, this book will also do the following:

- share a whole bunch of strategies for saving money both at the market every week and in the kitchen every day

- teach you how to build meals around naturally gluten-free foods and how to piggyback one dish off another to save time and money

- show you the basic foods and kitchen equipment that you really need (hint: there's not much) and give you advice on how to stock your kitchen with the ingredients that are the most versatile for gluten-free cooking

There are a few simple skills you can master that will dramatically expand your meal repertoire, and this book will share all of them. There is no need to get bored just because you're on a budget. Together, in this book, we'll make simple but delicious pancakes and blueberry muffins, soft pretzels and wontons, the perfect chocolate chip cookies and the ultimate in birthday cakes. Step by step, in the plain language of everyday home cooking, I'll show you how to make the comfort foods my family and I love, like chicken potpie and macaroni and cheese. You'll know how to bake a delicious apple pie when apples are abundant and even make your own fresh pasta—all gluten-free, all delicious and inexpensive.

I think you'll also be surprised when you learn how easy it is, with the right instruction and a little bit of practice, to make yeast breads, including never-fail white sandwich bread for packing everyone's lunches. Making

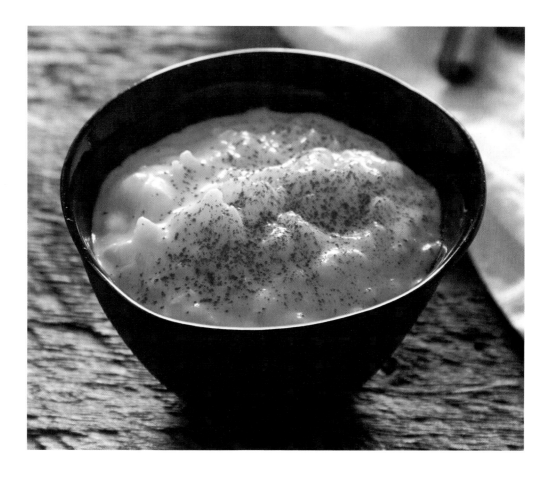

your own fresh bread is a uniquely joyful experience, and when you settle upon an all-purpose gluten-free flour blend you love, you'll be able to make everything in this book easily and on a budget. Some bake with a complicated bevy of exotic gluten-free flours, tweaking recipes here and there with a tablespoon of some flour I have never heard of before. When I go down that road, I always end up with remnants of flours in the wrong proportions, followed by a major bout of kitchen shyness, thinking I've lost my touch.

Trust me: stick with the basics, and you'll feel more confident and competent, both about your budget and about the way that kitchen of yours hums. You'll be amazed how much more enjoyable life is when you simplify how you cook and how your family eats. Never underestimate the power of kitchen confidence.

Remember: Life is sweet and fun. Gluten is expendable.

Love,

Nicole

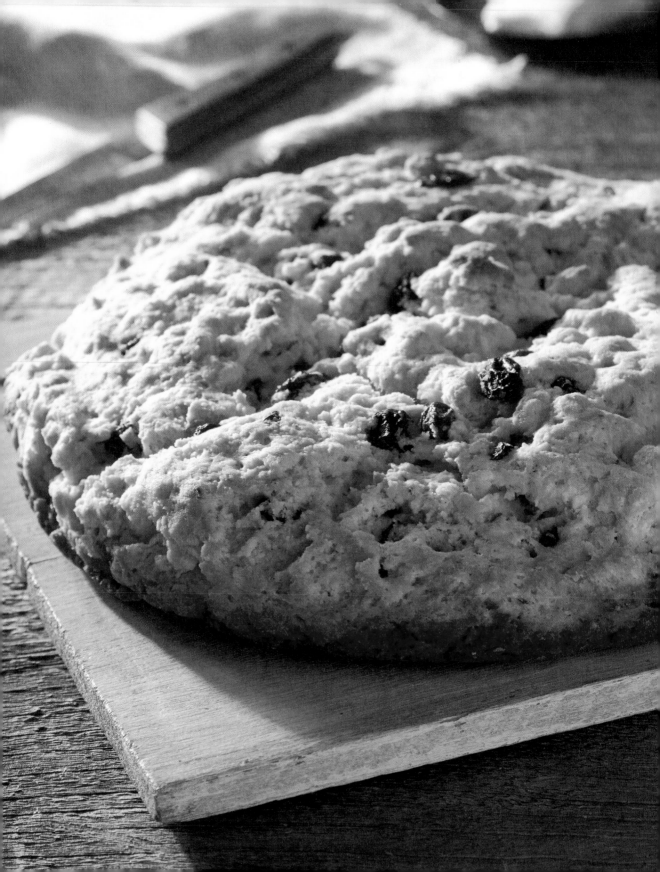

# SHOESTRING STRATEGIES: SAVING *at the* STORE *and in* YOUR KITCHEN

ALTHOUGH I WAS NEVER A SPEND-THRIFT, SAVING MONEY WASN'T ALWAYS SECOND NATURE TO ME. I was by no means born with a budget mindset, but by necessity, I earned it. So I understand that, until a shoestring mentality (to coin a phrase) becomes second nature, it can seem like a chore and even a burden to pay attention to saving money. You may even assume that the savings are not worth the effort. But if you're shopping for gluten-free ingredients, it's worth the effort—and that's where this book comes in.

Plain and simple, prepared gluten-free specialty foods are expensive. In fact, the *Canadian Journal of Dietetic Practice and Research* reported that gluten-free foods can cost nearly 250 percent more than conventional foods. If you're newly gluten-free, you're probably still suffering from sticker shock. One day, you're spending a modest $2.50 for a loaf of bread at the supermarket, and the next you're paying $8 or more for a gluten-free version. Or you go from paying $1.99 for a whole box of chocolate chip cookies to paying $7 for a tiny package of just six. At first, you may simply be thankful that gluten-free breads and cookies are readily available these days, whatever the cost. There can be a real sense of loss when you go gluten-free, and these packaged gluten-free foods may seem like a life raft. It's not that they necessarily taste so terrific (and often they don't), it's just that going gluten-free can seem so overwhelming, and many of us aren't accustomed to making things like a loaf of bread from scratch at home anyhow. The idea of relearning how to cook a whole new way can feel like a tall order. So it may seem easier

to turn to gluten-free packaged foods, no matter the cost—and that's where your food budget takes an unexpected turn for the worse.

I believe there's a different and better way. In this book, I will demystify the process and teach you how to make a big difference in the way you cook and in the way your family eats, with just a modest shift in perspective. You'll be eating fresh, homemade gluten-free foods that warm your home and your heart with a feeling of pride, give you a well-earned sense of accomplishment, and leave you with more money in your pocket at the end of the day. In this chapter, you'll learn a few meal-planning and money-saving strategies, and after that, I'll help you stock your pantry so that a savory and satisfying gluten-free meal for the whole family is at your fingertips every night of the week. Soon you won't need to rely upon a stockpile of overpriced, frozen gluten-free meals and desserts when you feel like you're out of fresh food (or ideas). You really won't run out of either for quite some time.

So let's begin. Here are nine ways you can start saving right away.

## TIP #1: USE COUPONS

To illustrate how far I've come, you should know that my husband's people are coupon people. They go way back. OK, I don't really know how far back they go, but I have firsthand evidence as far back as my father-in-law, and his practice borders on the obsessive. By contrast, for most of my life, I thought that "double coupons" at the market meant that you could use two coupons for the same item at the same time. Reasonable enough, I thought. For the still uninitiated, when a market accepts double coupons, it actually means that they will double your coupons, giving you twice the savings indicated on the coupon. How could I have seen that one coming? If the thought had occurred to me, I would have cast it aside, assuming it was arrogance to expect such royal treatment.

Coupons are no longer limited only to the Sunday newspaper variety. There are lots of other ways to use coupons to bring your gluten-free budget back down to earth. Here are a few of my secrets:

## Online Coupon Sites

There are websites like www.coupons.com and www.redplum.com that allow you to select and print coupons for a variety of mainstream brands. You're not likely to find many gluten-free specialty brands, but you will find many naturally gluten-free products. On the specialty side of things, there's www.mambosprouts.com. This is the company that produces those little coupon books that you often find in health-food stores and places like Whole Foods Market. Their website has printable coupons for many organic and health-food brands, which means there's usually some gluten-free products in the mix.

These days, many online shopping retailers carry a number of gluten-free products. Those products regularly go on sale, and the retailers, such as Vitacost, often have site-wide coupons that you can use for any purchase. A great source for online coupon codes is www.retailmenot.com. Whenever I'm purchasing anything online and there's a space for a coupon code in the checkout process, I

check RetailMeNot to see if it has a current coupon code. Often, it does.

## Supermarket Websites

Most major supermarkets have areas on their websites dedicated to helping you save money. You'll typically find the weekly circular, plus printable coupons from manufacturers and sometimes from the store itself. Some markets even have e-coupons that you can store on your frequent-shopper card. You can even store your savings cards electronically on your phone with the free CardStar app.

## Company Websites

Sometimes the best way to find coupons is to go directly to the source. Visit the websites of the companies that make the products you use, and you'll see that many of them have printable coupons right there. And be sure to check the sites for a place to register for promotions and discounts. Sometimes I fill out an online comment form and ask if the company would be willing to send me some coupons. You'd be surprised how many oblige.

Here are a few examples of company websites that offer coupons:

Arrowhead Mills (flours):
www.arrowheadmills.com/content/coupon-savings

Blue Diamond (almond milk, gluten-free crackers, nuts):
www.bluediamond.com/index.cfm?navid=8

Crunchmaster (gluten-free crackers):
www.crunchmaster.com/ppccoupon.aspx

Horizon Dairy:
www.horizon.com/signup

Land O'Lakes (great for savings on butter, eggs, cheese):
www.landolakes.com/offers/

Silk Soymilk:
https://silk.com/signup

Stonyfield Farm (yogurt):
www.stonyfield.com/register/

Udi's Gluten Free Foods:
http://shop.udisglutenfree.com/special-offers

## TIP #2: PRACTICE ONCE-A-WEEK COOKING

In the first chapter of recipes (see page 25), I'll introduce you to rudimentary recipes for simple but deliciously pitch-perfect stock, doughs, crusts, sauces, and other basics. To that end, I stock my refrigerator every single week with what I consider the building blocks of a week's worth of tasty gluten-free dinners: Pizza Dough (see page 36), Scratch Black Beans (see page 28), Fresh Pasta Dough (see page 35), Chicken Stock (see page 26), ground beef cooked with onions and garlic, and cooked brown rice.

To the pizza dough and cooked ground beef, simply add tomato sauce, grated cheese, and chopped frozen broccoli; you'll have a complete meal on the table in less than thirty minutes. The black beans are great for a quick (and super healthy) meal of rice and beans with Easy Enchilada Sauce (see page 45) or an incredibly flavorful black bean soup when simmered with some chicken stock.

You will need to commit to cooking—eating gluten-free on the cheap means you'll be cooking from scratch—but you won't need to be tethered to the kitchen, toiling daily for hours. There's no need, however, to go to the extreme of cooking an entire week's worth of dinners and desserts on the weekend—and then sleepwalking through the rest of the week. Keeping these basics on hand is how I avoid that kind of living. I make most of my basics on two days of the week, usually Sunday and either Tuesday or Wednesday. That way, they're always fresh and accessible.

## TIP #3: PRACTICE ONCE-A-MONTH COOKING

In addition to stocking the refrigerator once or twice a week, about once a month I create a few meals that are just one or two steps away from completion. Then I store them in the freezer. For example:

1. I often make Macaroni and Cheese (see page 165), pour it into a 13 × 9-inch baking dish, cover it, and freeze it until I'm ready to use it. Then, I just defrost it in the refrigerator during the day and bake it at night for dinner.

2. I make extra Potato Gnocchi (see page 137), freeze them in one even layer on a rimmed baking sheet, and then place them in a resealable freezer bag and boil them when I'm ready.

3. I shape raw Chocolate Chip Cookie dough (see page 199) into a cylinder, freeze it, and then I have slice-and-bake cookies whenever I need them.

4. I make and shape Buttermilk or Sweet Potato Biscuits or Drop Biscuits (see pages 103–108) and freeze them in a single layer while still raw, and then bake them when I need them.

5. Dinner Rolls (see page 99) also turn out very well if you bake them at 300°F until just set, and then cool and freeze them. When you're ready to use them, just pop them in a hot oven for about 5 to 7 minutes before serving.

Many other recipes lend themselves to being frozen after preparation but before baking. Examples that you'll find here in *Gluten-Free on a Shoestring* include:

Classic Apple Pie (see page 249)

Apple-Cinnamon Toaster Pastries (see page 72)

Beef Potstickers (see page 175)

Berry Scones (see page 81)

Easy Enchilada Sauce (see page 45)

Graham Crackers (see page 222)

Spinach Pie (see page 146)

And remember that breads like White Sandwich Bread (see page 109), Brioche Bread (see page 114), and English Muffin Bread (see page 113) freeze very well after they're baked and cooled. Simply slice the bread after it's cooled, and then wrap very tightly and freeze. Defrost one slice at a time in the toaster.

With nothing more than a well-conceived but flexible routine of cooking and preparation, you can greatly reduce your food budget and spending, eat better gluten-free foods, and enjoy yourself in the process.

## TIP #4: PIGGYBACK YOUR MEALS

Next, learn to piggyback one meal upon another to make the most of basic ingredients, which in turn allows you to buy loads of whatever happens to be in season and on sale at the market without allowing anything to go to waste. This concept is actually the basis of most good meal-planning services. Here are some examples of this idea at work: When you're rolling out pizza dough to make pizza, roll out a little extra for Beef Potpie (see page 186). If you're making polenta for Polenta Pizza (see page 157), make Tomato Polenta (see page 154). Lo Mein (see page 171), Szechuan Meatballs (see page 172), and Beef Potstickers (see page 175) all go well with Hoisin Sauce (see page 47). With this in mind, I'll make a double batch of the sauce and serve those three meals in the same week. If you have made three or four quarts of Chicken Stock (see page 26), use it in place of water to cook more flavorful brown rice. You can also use it to make Tortilla Soup (see page 191), Lemon Chicken (see page 179), Crispy Asian-Style Tofu (see page 150), Pot Roast (see page 192), or perhaps some Tomato Soup (see page 160). When in doubt, wrap something old and commonplace (like a chicken breast) in something new and exciting (like Savory Pastry Crust [see page 32]). Works every time.

I do my best to make at least a loose meal plan each week to take care of weeknight dinners because it makes my life easier and it makes meal piggybacking simple to do. Saturdays always seem kind of ad hoc, and since I cook so many basics on Sundays, dinner evolves quite naturally and always has a special dessert, like Chocolate Sandwich Cookies (see page 220) or a delicious Classic Apple Pie (see page 249).

For example, my week's menu might look like this:

1. **Monday:** Tortilla Soup (see page 191) with Dinner Rolls (see page 99), Rice Pudding (see page 257) for dessert (pudding made on Sunday and chilled overnight, rolls from my freezer stash, soup simmering in the evening while I get other things done around the house).

2. **Tuesday:** Sliced Meatlove (see page 168) with Barbecue Sauce (see page 47) on sliced bread, for example, White Sandwich Bread (see page 109) or Brioche Bread (see page 114), and side salad (double recipe of Meatlove made this evening, half frozen for use on Thursday, bread from freezer stock).

3. **Wednesday:** Scratch Black Bean (see page 28) and cheese burritos with chopped, defrosted frozen broccoli, served with brown rice (black beans made on Sunday, Flour Tortillas [see page 121] made this evening).

4. **Thursday:** Meatballs and tomato sauce over gluten-free spaghetti with Dinner Rolls and defrosted frozen spinach sautéed in garlic and oil (meatballs made from Meatlove defrosted in the refrigerator overnight, rolls defrosted from freezer stash and warmed in a 350°F oven, spinach defrosted and sautéed before serving).

5. **Friday:** Who doesn't love pizza?! Pizza dough (see page 36) made earlier in the week, rolled out and baked tonight, topped with defrosted frozen broccoli, defrosted frozen spinach, slices of

tomato, and/or browned ground beef and sautéed onions.

If any gluten-free bread goes stale (gasp!), make Bread Pudding (see page 88). Bananas browning too quickly? Make Banana Pancake Muffins (see page 68) or even freeze them whole and unpeeled. Then when you need to use those bananas, just microwave them for about thirty seconds to soften before baking. Potatoes starting to go bad? Make a Tortilla Española (see page 60). Cupboards bare? But then you notice you have lots of milk on hand, and you know there's some cornmeal in the back of your pantry. Make Cornmeal Spoonbread (see page 153) and serve it with some black beans. Apples starting to show their age? Maybe you went apple picking and, like me, an extra bag seemed like a great idea while you were in the orchard. It's another story when you get home. Make a quick applesauce by peeling, coring, and slicing the apples and putting them in a heavy-bottom saucepan with sugar and ground cinnamon to taste and a little water to prevent the apples from burning. Even better, make an Apple Crisp (page 253), which is nearly as simple to make as applesauce.

**Check the freezer.** If you have a lot of frozen spinach, make a quick Spinach Pie (page 146): no excuses—that Savory Olive Oil Crust (see page 33) doesn't need to rise, so it's ready in a snap. Just poke around your refrigerator, freezer, and pantry. There's plenty there to satisfy everyone.

## TIP #6: BE SMART ABOUT HOW YOU STORE YOUR FOOD

*Prevention* magazine advises storing onions and potatoes in the refrigerator but separately, since the moisture in the potatoes will cause the onions to age faster. They'll last longer, and as an added bonus, those cold onions give off fewer fumes when you cut them. Easier on the wallet, easier on those tender eyes of yours. Store your all-purpose gluten-free flour in an airtight container on your counter or in your pantry, unless you don't plan to use it all in one year's time, in which case you should store it in the refrigerator. If possible, store apples in a separate crisper, away from other foods, since they can rot other foods faster. If you're using reduced-sodium gluten-free soy sauce or tamari, store it in the refrigerator because it will spoil faster than its full-sodium counterpart. Store eggs on the bottom shelf, in the container you bought them in, and keep that container closed so the odors of other foods don't mingle with your eggs.

## TIP #7: IF IT'S ON SALE, BUY IN BULK

When potatoes of any kind are on sale, stock up and make Oven Hash Brown Quiche (see page 63), Potato Gnocchi (see page 137), Shepherd's Pie (see page 185), and Tomato Soup (see page 160).

In addition to buying some items online (see page 14), you can also lower your gluten-free spending by just buying whatever essentials you can find at your regular supermarket. Check the circular that lists store specials from at least one market every week. Certain cooking staples, like unsalted butter quarters and ricotta cheese, are on sale pretty often. Be sure to use the store's loyalty or club card to get the savings without having to use any coupons. When items like these are on sale, stock up. Just check the sell-by and use-by dates carefully and reach toward the back of the grocer's dairy case for the newest products. Butter frequently has a very long shelf life and can also be frozen and used after the date stamped on the packaging. (Just trust your nose. When dairy is spoiled, it smells spoiled.)

## TIP #8: GROW A VEGETABLE GARDEN

Even better than smart shopping and buying produce when it's on sale, plant a garden when the weather allows in your area and grow your own bell peppers. Whatever the climate, with few exceptions, growing your own vegetables can be a very smart way to defray the high cost of buying produce.

But even so, there are some vegetables, like carrots and celery, that are so inexpensive to buy fresh in the market that I do not ever grow my own. Then there are those vegetables that are far superior when grown fresh and thrive so readily that it's silly not to try your hand at growing your own. Tomatoes, zucchini, and cucumbers come to mind. Speaking of cucumbers, why is it that even in the middle of the summer where I live, I can't remember the last time I saw a cucumber on sale for less than seventy-five cents each? I'm thinking about opening up a small farm stand in front of my house. In my spare time. Seventy-five cents for one cucumber is highway robbery!

## TIP #9: BUY FROZEN VEGGIES

Don't worry. If the very thought of growing your own vegetables is making your palms sweat, don't let it slow you down. Forget the garden. During most of the year, I use frozen vegetables. They're frozen at the peak of freshness and typically cost heaps less than their fresh counterparts. A one-pound bag of good-quality frozen broccoli crowns runs me less than $2, and there's no waste. One pound of fresh broccoli, on sale, will cost at least $2.50, it takes up a ton of space in my refrigerator, and preparing it is much more labor intensive. Frozen vegetables are ready whenever and in whatever quantity you need them, and they don't spoil for ages. Use frozen, buy fresh when it's on sale, and keep on keepin' on.

# WHAT *to* BUY *and* FROM WHERE

BUYING WHOLE FOODS, GLUTEN-FREE OR NOT, CAN BE EXPENSIVE—BUT IT DOESN'T HAVE TO BE IF YOU follow a few straightforward guidelines. In these recipes, I will walk you through how to make good use of whole-food ingredients to create delicious, satisfying foods that everyone will love. But first things first.

We'll start with the proper contents of a well-stocked, gluten-free pantry, the backbone of your kitchen. These are the items that you're bound to use on a regular basis, so it's always money well spent. You don't have to buy them every week. You just have to keep them in stock because they make everything else possible. Then we'll go through what to buy at the market and online on a regular basis. Finally, we'll review the basic kitchen equipment that you'll need (hint: it isn't much). Think of these everyday basics like good, clean underwear. You wouldn't carefully select a beautiful outfit (here, a great recipe), one that makes you feel like a million bucks, only to wear it over a pair of granny panties that give you unsightly panty lines and keep you tugging at them all day, would you? Of course not. Carefully select just the right basic food items, and you can rock any recipe in your kitchen.

Our pantry items in place, we'll move on to clever strategies for choosing which perishable foods to buy every week and for getting the most out of your weekly trip to the market.

## THE WELL-STOCKED, GLUTEN-FREE, SHOESTRING-FRIENDLY PANTRY

Do you know any home cooks who seem to throw together a dinner with what seems like little to no planning? Cooks who can effortlessly accommodate a few more guests at the last minute without simply adding some more water to thin the soup? These cooks know how to keep their pantries well stocked, and they're confident in their own kitchens. This can be you! Updating your pantry with essential, all-purpose items is your first step toward the good, gluten-free life, and it's within reach.

When you always have on hand what you need to prepare meals (and don't have to reinvent the wheel every time you need to write a shopping list), you'll be much less tempted to order takeout, rely on frozen gluten-free pizzas, or grab those pricey packages of gluten-free cupcakes. In my kitchen, I don't stock store-bought sauces and dressings. Instead, I stock the ingredients that serve as the bases for those sauces and dressings. I don't stock ready-made pie shells, but I do stock the ingredients I need to make basic sweet and savory piecrusts. I make dough for each type and freeze it in portions. I always have the ingredients on hand to make last-minute cupcakes and frosting ("I forgot to tell you there's a birthday party in school tomorrow, Mom!") and perfect chocolate chip cookies. Remember, I even make my own slice-and-bake cookie dough, shaped into a log and frozen for just such an emergency.

Now, let's take a look at what you should expect to buy on a regular basis. The following items are the ingredients that should have a constant presence in your cupboard, refrigerator, or freezer, as the case may be. You may already have most of these items right now and just need to supplement with a few more to round things out. If you don't have many of these staples, you will have to stock up, and there will be an up-front cost. But this is an investment, as essential to the proper functioning of your kitchen as the sink and stove. And like any good investment, over time it will pay off—day after day, meal after meal. Count on it.

PANTRY STAPLES

## Oil, Vinegar, and Condiments

- Extra-virgin olive oil
- Canola oil (or other neutral vegetable oil)
- Sesame oil
- Nonstick cooking spray (most are gluten-free, but be a savvy consumer)
- White wine vinegar
- Balsamic vinegar (regular or white)
- Apple cider vinegar
- Rice vinegar
- Gluten-free soy sauce or tamari
- Worcestershire sauce (check to make sure the brand is gluten-free)

## Grocery

- Tomato paste (canned or in a tube)
- Canned tomato purée (my favorite brand is Cento)
- Honey
- Unsulfured molasses
- Pure maple syrup
- Peanut butter
- Mayonnaise
- Tahini (sesame paste)

## Beans, Pasta, and Grains

- Dried black beans
- Dried gluten-free pasta
- Gluten-free old-fashioned rolled oats (only buy certified gluten-free)
- Brown rice
- Short-grain rice (like arborio rice)
- Coarsely ground (yellow) cornmeal
- Polenta cornmeal (cornmeal especially milled for making polenta)
- Precooked cornmeal (masa harina corn flour)
- Quinoa flakes
- Gluten-free cornflake cereal

## Baking

- All-purpose gluten-free flour plus ingredients to make homemade all-purpose gluten-free flour blends (see page 21)
- Xanthan gum
- Cornstarch

- Expandex modified tapioca starch

- Whey protein isolate

- Superfine white rice flour

- Potato starch

- Tapioca starch/flour

- Baking powder

- Baking soda

- Instant yeast

- Brown sugar (light or dark)

- Confectioners' sugar

- Granulated sugar

- Unsweetened cocoa powder (Dutch-processed and natural)

- Semisweet chocolate chips

- Light coconut milk (canned)

- Low-fat evaporated milk (canned)

- Cream of tartar

- Vegetable shortening

- Pure vanilla extract

- Whole vanilla beans

## Seasonings

- Kosher salt

- Tablet(fine) salt

- Black peppercorns (for grinding)

- Ground cinnamon

- Dried oregano

- Dried parsley

- Ground cumin

- Chile flakes

- Chile powder

- Dried bay leaves

## Fruits and Nuts

- Whole cranberries

- Dried cranberries (unsweetened)

- Thompson raisins

- Sliced almonds

- Pecan pieces

## Frozen Vegetables

- Frozen peas

- Frozen broccoli crowns

- Frozen spinach (chopped or whole)

- Frozen corn kernels

## TO MARKET, TO MARKET: WHAT TO BUY WEEKLY AT THE GROCERY

Now that you have your pantry shopping list, here's a meal shopping list for a typical week cooking the *Gluten-Free on a Shoestring* way. Of course, this is a general list, and you can adapt it easily to accommodate any other dietary needs and restrictions you adhere to.

## Your Weekly Ingredient Shopping List

(Remember: Your regular pantry items are not included here.)

## Fresh Fruits and Vegetables

- Apples (Granny Smith, Golden Delicious, McIntosh, etc., especially in the fall when they're cheaper)

- Bananas

- Butternut squash

- Carrots

- Celery hearts

- Garlic

- Ginger root

- Leeks

- Lemons

- Potatoes (red and yellow, select potatoes of similar size for even cooking)

- Sweet potatoes

- Yellow onions

## Dairy Case

- Eggs

- Mozzarella cheese (or nondairy cheese)

- Cheddar cheese (or nondairy cheese)

- Part-skim ricotta cheese

- Unsalted butter (or nondairy, trans fat–free margarine)

- Low-fat milk (or nondairy milk, such as soy milk, nut milk, or rice milk)

- Extra-firm tofu

## Meat

- Bone-in, skin-on chicken thighs

- Bone-in, skin-on chicken breasts

- Boneless, skinless chicken breasts

- Lean ground beef

Now on to a few bits of advice about some foods used in these recipes:

**Eggs.** All of the recipes in this book that call for eggs provide a weight measurement for the eggs as weighed out of their shells. The weight provided per egg out of the shell is 50 grams, which corresponds to a large egg. I indicate the size by way of weight, rather than using the term *large*, to enable readers who have nonstandard eggs to use whatever eggs they like. If your egg doesn't weigh approximately 50 grams out of the shell, simply add more beaten egg until the proper weight is reached. (For more on buying a kitchen scale, see page 16.)

**Cheese.** I often buy certain cheeses, such as Parmesan, in blocks and grate as I go. With other cheeses, like mozzarella, I often buy them already grated (as with anything already prepared and packaged, carefully check labels and ingredients to ensure that the product is gluten-free). Although my general rule is not to pay someone else to do something that you could do easily for yourself, this is a notable exception. Buying grated cheese is frequently less expensive than buying a block of cheese, believe it or not. Plus, a package of grated cheese has a longer life in your refrigerator than a block of cheese does. And there is nothing more expensive than spoiled food that must be disposed of.

**Fresh fruits and vegetables.** The same rule of thumb applies to fresh produce, especially fruit. I look at it this way: if I know that fruit is going to be eaten within a week, I am happy to go out of my way to a produce-only market that sells fruits and vegetables that are a few days old and much less expensive. But if there's a chance that it won't all be eaten in a week or less, it is more cost effective to spend a bit more on the very freshest produce, if it is available where you live. If you do buy produce that has aged a few days, be sure to buy only what you know you will use straightaway. Remember the rule about spoiled food: if you end up having to throw it away, you haven't saved anything.

Buy bananas that are bright yellow with a hint of green, and try to buy them in a place that sells them by the banana, not by weight. You'll find it's a better deal—and you can pick the largest bananas from the bunch.

**Buy the produce that is currently in season.** If you are able to shop in a large market, you will find all fruits year-round. But in the case of off-season produce, like berries in the winter, what you'll find will be almost universally much more expensive and much less tasty. They also tend to spoil more quickly. Buy berries all summer, wait to buy stone fruit like peaches, plums, and nectarines in the late summer, and stock up on apples in the fall, and you won't be sorry. There are some exceptions, like grapes that are flown in from around the world and are good quality all year (and are always on sale somewhere) and hothouse tomatoes that are always good (but only buy them on sale or they'll be way too expensive). Start turning your attention to what seems plentiful during a particular season, and you'll be glad you did. For those of you in the United States, this site will tell you, by state, what is in season each month of the year: www.sustainabletable.org /seasonalfoodguide/.

**Dairy items.** Only in a real pinch should you have to pay full price for mainstream market items like butter, cheese, and milk, since they so regularly go on sale. When milk is on sale, it is often a loss leader, so the store may actually be selling it below cost to lure you into the store with the hope that you'll buy other items at full price (which, of course, you won't, but they don't know that).

**Meat.** Meats also tend to go on sale at the market pretty regularly and often at a steep discount. Buy some extra, and freeze what you can't use right away. Don't buy too much, though, or you won't remember to use it. Buy larger family packs of meat, unwrap the package at home, use what you can right away, and freeze the rest in airtight packaging, labeling the package with the date. And just like the grocer does, rotate perishable items in your refrigerator, making sure the freshest foods are on top and easily within reach.

## ORDERING ONLINE

In recent years, the number and availability of gluten-free products have expanded dramatically. Everyday supermarkets now carry all-purpose gluten-free flours, and some even have dedicated natural or organic food sections with gluten-free products. There are also stores like Trader Joe's and Whole Foods that carry a nice selection of gluten-free products and often even carry their own line of certified gluten-free products. That's the good news.

But not everyone has access to these stores. Generally speaking, online retailers still offer a much broader selection of gluten-free products and ingredients. Plus, if you're smart about the way you order online, you can stretch your gluten-free budget. Here are a few ideas.

## 1. Order Your Flours Online

As I mentioned, you can find certain brands of all-purpose gluten-free flour in many supermarkets and specialty stores. But remember, you're going to be using a lot of gluten-free flour, so buying it in one-pound, retail-size bags is not very shoestring friendly. You need a better solution.

Over the years, I have used many brands of all-purpose gluten-free flour, and my favorite overall gluten-free flour is Better Batter Gluten Free Flour (www.betterbatter .org). Better Batter works very well in all of my recipes that call for an all-purpose gluten-free flour. It's also free of all other major allergens. The ingredients as listed are rice flour, brown rice flour, potato starch, potato flour, pectin (lemon derivative), and xanthan gum.

There are many things that really make this brand stand out. For starters, as noted above, the flour blend already incorporates xanthan gum, which happens to be one of the more expensive gluten-free baking ingredients. Score. (Just be sure to omit the xanthan gum ingredient from the recipes in this book if you are using Better Batter or any other all-purpose gluten-free flour blend that contains xanthan gum as part of the premade blend.) On top of that, you can order Better Batter in bulk at a reduced rate. Best of all, the company typically offers reasonable shipping rates. This last point is especially important. If you've ever ordered heavy items like flour or mixes online, you know how those shipping charges can really add up. So when you do the math, Better Batter is a winner.

You'll need to purchase the component flours for the Basic Gum-Free Gluten-Free Flour blend (see page 21) online. I find that Vitacost (www.vitacost.com) often has the best price. Sign up for their e-mails to receive notification of specials. You'll need superfine white rice flour, which is made by Authentic Foods and available through Vitacost. Amazon.com also carries Authentic Foods flours. Vitacost makes its own proprietary brand of so-called superfine white rice flour. It is more finely ground than many but not nearly as finely ground as Authentic Foods.

If you choose to build an all-purpose gluten-free flour blend (see page 21), you'll need all of the individual flours as listed in the blends. Bob's Red Mill products are fine for corn products, like polenta corn grits, coarsely ground yellow cornmeal, and even masa harina corn flour. However, none of their all-purpose gluten-free flour blends will work in my recipes. I have found that they are of very inconsistent quality. Their rice flours are very grainy, and I avoid them completely. You must use superfine rice flours when building a blend, or your baked goods will suffer greatly.

Please see a full discussion about building your own all-purpose gluten-free flour and other blends for use in the recipes in this book later in this chapter.

## 2. Save with Amazon.com

I love Amazon.com for gluten-free shopping, and there are several reasons why I think you will, too. Amazon carries many gluten-free items, including well-known brands like Barilla Gluten Free Pasta, Arrowhead Mills, Authentic Foods flours, Erewhon Natural Foods, Nature's Path Organic (including EnviroKidz Organic), Amy's Kitchen, Annie's Homegrown, Glutino, and many more. Prices are generally very good, and items are often sold in money-saving multipacks. We like multipacks. Also, the majority of Amazon items qualify for free shipping if you join Amazon Prime. This is a huge advantage over many specialty gluten-free online retailers.

On top of the good prices and the free shipping, certain Amazon.com products also qualify for the Subscribe & Save program. This subscription service works like this: you sign up and agree to get repeat shipments of your item at a monthly interval you choose. When you do, you get a percentage off the initial order and all the subsequent ones. The best part is, you can suspend or cancel the subscription at any time, and you will still get the money off your original order.

### 3. Sign Up for E-Mail Alerts and Newsletters

For selection, you can't beat online retailers like Gluten Free Delivers (http://glutenfree delivers.com/) and Gluten Free Mall (www .glutenfreemall.com). Visit these sites and sign up for their free e-mail alerts. If you don't mind getting some extra e-mail, it's worth it. You'll probably receive special offers and discount codes, often for 10 percent off your order. I usually find something of value.

#### THE BEST GLUTEN-FREE VALUES AND THE BEST PLACES TO FIND THEM

When you shop smart, you really can extend your food budget. And these savings can go a long way toward offsetting the pain of the extra money we simply must spend on certain gluten-free staples, such as dried gluten-free pasta and all-purpose gluten free flour (which are typically more expensive than the gluten-containing varieties).

I recommend buying gluten-free flour, gluten-free pasta, gluten-free cereal, cornmeal, xanthan gum, and certified gluten-free oats online. At the grocery store, buy raw meat and chicken, milk and cream, butter, eggs, cheese, dried beans, rice, tomato sauce, produce, and frozen vegetables. At a warehouse club, buy baking staples like sugar, baking chips, honey, molasses, salt, produce (when possible, as it's usually very fresh so it keeps well), olive oil, vinegars, gluten-free tamari or soy sauce, Worcestershire sauce, dried herbs and spices, and rice and dried beans when possible.

#### ESSENTIAL KITCHEN EQUIPMENT

Finally, let's discuss the equipment you'll need to keep things humming along nicely. A well-equipped kitchen by my standards is one that has an oven in working order, an oven thermometer (most ovens are improperly calibrated and the temperatures are off by quite a lot, so let an oven thermometer be your guide), a stovetop with at least one or two burners in working order, a refrigerator, a sink, and some counter space. It doesn't take much. There are, however, a few pieces of equipment that I consider to be money well spent if not entirely essential to a well-appointed kitchen. Remember, you are going to be cooking all of your family's food in this kitchen of yours, and you'll be saving boat-loads of money in the process. You should have what you need to do it right.

## Kitchen Equipment

**Oven thermometer:** so important to proper functioning it bears repeating; average cost $15 or less.

**Digital kitchen scale:** essential for building a flour blend (see page 21) and for consistent baking results, including for weighing eggs; can cost as little as $15. (I had a basic Escali scale for many years—until I dropped it into a bowl of water!)

**Rimmed metal baking sheets:** quarter-sheet and half-sheet pans are particularly useful and fit in most any oven; Nordic Ware makes a great basic baking sheet.

**10- or 12-inch nonstick frying pan**

**Large (7½ quart) enamel cast-iron Dutch oven:** there are many companies that make good-quality enameled cast iron these days, including Martha Stewart brand. Cast iron in general heats quickly and evenly, despite the high-performance burners on my stove that tend toward the overzealous. And even stuck-on foods come off easily when you soak it in hot water and soap and then use Bar Keepers Friend, a mild abrasive cleanser that is very similar to Bon Ami.

**Large pasta pot:** plus a dedicated colander, if you use one—I often don't, since I'm too lazy to clean and dry it every time (colanders are so hard to dry).

**Medium heavy-bottom saucepan:** I have a stainless steel Cuisinart brand, and it wasn't cheap (about $75 at a Cuisinart outlet), but it's worth the money for its even cooking and easy cleanup.

**Springform pan:** no need to spend much on this item.

**Stand mixer:** if possible, buy a good one that will be a workhorse for you and stand the test of time.

**Food processor:** indispensable for making homemade hummus, grating or slicing large quantities of vegetables, and grinding whole cuts of meat. You can usually get away with one of those very economical miniature Cuisinart food processors and just work in batches.

**Immersion blender:** an inexpensive item—read: don't pay more than $30, give or take—that will earn its keep in just a few uses.

**Asian-style spider strainer:** a cheap-o item.

**Cutting boards:** my favorite brand is Epicurean, as the cutting boards don't dull knives, are dishwasher safe, and last forever.

**Chef's knife or Santoku knife:** I have a Wüsthof Classic 7-inch Santoku knife, which is a great all-purpose knife, and I like the way it feels in my hand. It cost about $85, and I bought it years ago and sharpen it somewhat regularly. If you're having trouble deciding which style and which brand to buy, try going to a chef's store or the knife department of a large department store and speak to a salesperson. They're very knowledgeable.

**Serrated carving knife:** I have a Wüsthof but for no particular reason. This knife won't be used nearly as much as the all-purpose chef's or Santoku knife, so you don't need to break the bank on it, but for slicing all those loaves of gluten-free bread you're going to be turning out, nothing else comes close to a Wüsthof large serrated carving knife.

**Small paring knife:** I have both a Zyliss and a Wüsthof; neither was very expensive. No need to spend much on this type of knife, but you do need it.

**Large, flat, high heat–resistant silicone spatula:** please, no plastic or it will melt; no metal or it will scratch everything.

**High heat–resistant silicone slotted spatula:** again, no plastic or metal, please.

**Vegetable peeler:** any will do.

**Pastry brush:** I have a silicone one because I like that it's heat resistant.

**Measuring spoons and cups:** any will do.

**Wooden or silicone spoons:** silicone will keep very, very well.

**Metal balloon whisks:** for whisking in bowls.

**Flat whisk:** for whisking in pots and pans.

**Rolling pin:** I like the French kind, without handles; the ones with handles just seem to spin and spin.

A word about preventing cross-contamination of gluten-free foods in your kitchen: don't make your life any harder than it has to be. Each time I hear a tale of a household cooking one meal for the only celiac in the family and one for everyone else in the family—either out of fear that the gluten-free food is not going to be palatable to the non-celiacs or because of the excessive cost of the gluten-free meal—I shed one sad, lonely tear. Make delicious, reasonably priced gluten-free food, make a lot of it, and invite the neighbors over. Go ahead, host Thanksgiving. I promise you, your family and your guests won't know the difference (except that maybe it'll be better than last year's).

To the extent that you must cook and bake any conventional, gluten-containing foods, be careful. Gluten is sticky. Use a dedicated colander for gluten-free pastas, and don't even consider using a strainer that has seen the likes of gluten in its lifetime. Put everything you can in the dishwasher, and when you're preparing, cooking, baking, or serving gluten-free foods, avoid using anything porous (like wood or plastic utensils, cutting boards, or storage containers) that once contained or was used to prepare gluten-containing foods. Exercise caution when reusing basically anything that has lots of grooves and crevices that tend to hold onto crumbs, like nonstick muffin tins and springform pans. That advice about only cooking and baking gluten-free is starting to look better and better, right?

### IF YOU'RE DAIRY-FREE, TOO

I get lots of questions about whether dairy-free substitutions can be made in recipes, and the answer is almost always yes. Every recipe in this book that calls for a dairy-containing ingredient can handle a dairy-free substitute, except where specifically noted otherwise. And the vast majority handle the substitution very well (with the exception of the bread flour for the newer bread recipes, see page 21).

In my house, we were dairy-free for a spell a number of years ago, and we did it for long enough that I did develop some allegiance to specific brands of two particular products: cheese and a butter alternative. After trying what seemed like scores of dairy-free, gluten-free cheeses, the one that won my heart was, well, Follow Your Heart brand Vegan Gourmet cheese alternatives. It not only says that it melts, but it does, in fact, melt. Sure, it melts a bit better in the microwave than in the oven, but it's simple enough to work around a little quirk like that. It comes in a block, and it even grates nicely. Many other brands, like Daiya, Field Roast Chao, and Treeline Treenut Cheese (made from cashews), are available, and there are also many recipes for making homemade vegan cheeses.

My choice for a gluten-free, dairy-free butter alternative is butter-flavored Spectrum brand nonhydrogenated vegetable oil. Earth Balance brand vegan buttery sticks, like margarine, contain a significant amount of moisture. They're fine for cooking but not a proper substitute for most baking, particularly when the butter in the ingredient list is meant to be kept cold, as in pastries and biscuits.

In all the other dairy-alternative product categories, like milk and sour cream, they all seem to work just fine. It's really a matter of taste. Just be sure to use an unflavored, unsweetened nondairy milk for cooking and baking, and avoid fat-free milks as they really taste like cloudy water.

## GLUTEN-FREE FLOUR BLENDS

### General Guidelines

In gluten-free baking, no one individual flour can serve as an "all-purpose" flour, one that functions largely the same as conventional gluten-containing all-purpose flour. Instead, we rely upon a blend of flours that together are good for "all purposes." Just like flours in conventional baking, no one blend is absolutely ideal for every unique purpose. A pastry flour is ideally low in protein and high in starch for a certain lightness and comparative lack of

chew. Bread flour is essentially the opposite: low starch, high protein for flexibility and chew. So it goes in gluten-free baking as well.

You can either purchase an all-purpose gluten-free flour, already blended, or mix your own for use in every recipe in this cookbook that calls for an all-purpose gluten-free flour. If you would like to purchase a ready-made all-purpose gluten-free flour blend, below are the two I recommend. If you would prefer to blend your own, there are recipes on page 21 for you to do just that.

When a recipe calls specifically for the Basic Gum-Free Gluten-Free Flour blend, only the specific amount of xanthan gum indicated as a separate ingredient in the recipe, if any, is appropriate. Those recipes require a lower xanthan gum proportion than other recipes, or none at all, and use of an all-purpose gluten-free flour blend that already contains xanthan gum will lead to a poor result.

### Commercially Available All-Purpose Gluten-Free Flours

Better Batter and Cup4Cup. These are my two favorite brands of commercially available all-purpose gluten-free flour blends. The two all-purpose gluten-free flour blend recipes I provide below are a Mock Better Batter All-Purpose Gluten-Free Flour, which approximates the results achieved with Better Batter Gluten Free Flour, and my Better Than Cup-4Cup All-Purpose Gluten-Free Flour, which corrects what I think is an imbalance in Cup-4Cup itself. Either of those blends can be used successfully in any recipes in this book that call for an all-purpose gluten- free flour.

Better Batter Gluten Free Flour is the

one true all-purpose gluten-free flour that I have used most consistently since 2009. It is a well-balanced blend of superfine white rice flour, superfine brown rice flour, tapioca starch, potato starch, potato flour, xanthan gum, and pectin. I always order it directly from the company itself through their website, betterbatter.org, as that is the best price, and find it cheaper (and of course more convenient) to purchase it than to build my own with individual flours. See page 15 for a more complete discussion of this particular blend.

Cup4Cup gluten-free flour really works best as a pastry flour or a cake flour, as it is quite high in starch, and I don't recommend it for best results in the recipes in this book as an all-purpose gluten-free flour.

**Cup4Cup as Cake Flour.** If you do decide to use Cup4Cup in any of the recipes in this book as an all-purpose gluten free-flour, if that recipe also calls for cornstarch, please use more Cup4Cup, gram for gram, in place of the cornstarch. Therefore, if a recipe calls for 100 grams of all-purpose gluten-free flour and 10 grams of cornstarch, if you are using Cup4Cup as the all-purpose gluten-free flour, instead use 110 grams of Cup4Cup.

## Specialty Gluten-Free Flours

**Expandex modified tapioca starch.** Expandex brand modified tapioca starch is a chemically (not genetically!) modified tapioca starch that, in small amounts and in the proper recipe, gives gluten-free baked goods an elasticity that can't be achieved otherwise. I first introduced this incredibly useful ingredient in *Gluten-Free on a Shoestring Bakes Bread*, and it remains irreplaceable in building my gluten-free bread flour

blend (see page 21). In certain, limited instances, however, Expandex can be replaced with plain tapioca starch/flour gram for gram. In this book, I have indicated this possibility in the recipes themselves. For additional information on where to buy Expandex modified tapioca starch, please see the Resources page on my blog: http://glutenfreeonashoestring.com. (You'll also find information on how to use Ultratex 3, another type of modified tapioca starch, in place of Expandex in the bread flour; Ultratex 3 is more widely available online worldwide and is approximately three times as strong as Expandex.)

**Gluten-free bread flour.** To build the bread flour blend on page 21, I use Now Whey Protein Isolate (which is nearly all protein—you must use isolate, not whey powder or whey protein concentrate), which I purchase online through Vitacost or Amazon, depending upon which site has the best price at that time. There is also a brand of whey protein isolate available on Amazon called Opportuniteas Grass-Fed Whey Protein Isolate that is cold processed using raw milk and is GMO-free, if that is important to you.

## The Homemade Flour Blends

All the flour blend recipes that follow can be multiplied by as many factors as you like. I typically make at least 10 cups at a time by just multiplying every ingredient by 10, placing the ingredients in a large, airtight, lidded container, and whisking very well. For an online calculator that does the math for you, please see the Flour Blends page on my website: http://glutenfreeonashoestring.com/all-purpose-gluten-free-flour-recipes/.

Large batches can be stored in sealed

containers at a cool room temperature. I store at least one 28-cup container of an all-purpose gluten-free flour in my pantry. It will be as fresh as the freshness dates on the component flours dictate.

## 1 CUP (140 G) MOCK BETTER BATTER ALL-PURPOSE GLUTEN-FREE FLOUR

42 grams (about ¼ cup) superfine white rice flour (30%)

42 grams (about ¼ cup) superfine brown rice flour (30%)

21 grams (about 2⅓ tablespoons) tapioca starch/flour (15%)

21 grams (about 2⅓ tablespoons) potato starch (15%)

7 grams (about 1¾ teaspoons) potato flour (5%)

4 grams (about 2 teaspoons) xanthan gum (3%)

3 grams (about 1½ teaspoons) pure powdered fruit pectin (2%)

## 1 CUP (140 G) BETTER THAN CUP4CUP ALL-PURPOSE GLUTEN-FREE FLOUR

43 grams (about ¼ cup) superfine white rice flour (31%)

25 grams (about 8⅓ teaspoons) cornstarch (18%)

24 grams (about 2½ tablespoons) superfine brown rice flour (17%)

21 grams (about 2⅓ tablespoons) tapioca starch/flour (15%)

20 grams (about 3⅓ tablespoons, before grinding) nonfat dry milk, ground into a finer powder (14%)

4 grams (about 1 teaspoon) potato starch (3%)

3 grams (about 1½ teaspoons) xanthan gum (2%)

## 1 CUP (140 G) BASIC GUM-FREE GLUTEN-FREE FLOUR

92 grams (about 8¾ tablespoons) superfine white rice flour (66%)

31 grams (about 3¼ tablespoons) potato starch (22%)

17 grams (about 5 teaspoons) tapioca starch/flour (12%)

## 1 CUP (140 G) GLUTEN-FREE BREAD FLOUR

100 grams (about 11½ tablespoons) Mock Better Batter All-Purpose Gluten-Free Flour (71%)

25 grams (about 5 tablespoons) unflavored whey protein isolate (18%)

15 grams (about 5 teaspoons) Expandex modified tapioca starch (11%)

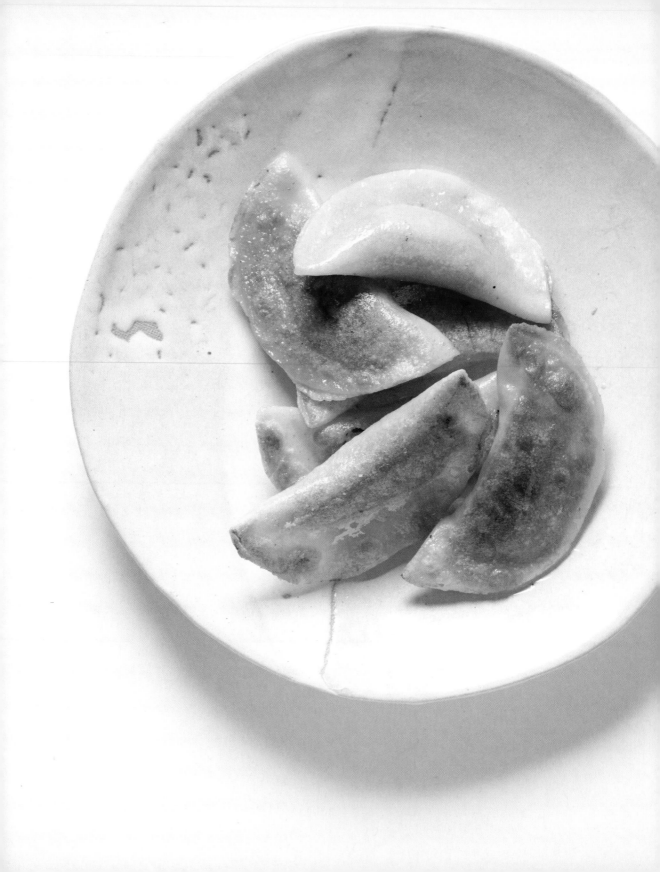

# KITCHEN CONFIDENCE: BASIC RECIPES THAT SERVE *as the* FOUNDATION *for* MANY OTHERS

# MEAL INGREDIENTS

# CHICKEN STOCK

*Makes* 2 quarts (or 8 cups) stock

THIS IS A BIG ONE. THE RECIPES IN THIS BOOK ARE AWASH IN CHICKEN STOCK AS AN ingredient. Where I live, it's common to find prepared gluten-free chicken stock on the shelf of even the smaller grocery chains, and I use it frequently. It's just so handy and versatile. I don't always make homemade stock myself, but when I do, it's always better. And of course there's the cost savings, when a single box of good-quality chicken stock like Pacific brand is typically at least $2.50. When I make stock myself, my family and I eat the chicken and all of the vegetables we cooked to make the broth, so it's like we're getting the stock for free. And if I leave the vegetables in the stock and just remove the chicken and the bay leaf and purée with an immersion blender, it's a wonderfully rich base for Chicken and Dumplings Soup (see page 188).

4 skin-on, bone-in chicken thighs

2 carrots, cut into 1-inch chunks

2 stalks of celery, cut into 1-inch chunks

1 large yellow onion, peeled and quartered

6 to 8 garlic cloves, whole with skin removed

1 butternut squash, peeled, seeded, and cut into large chunks

1 dried bay leaf

2 tablespoons (36 g) kosher salt

1 teaspoon freshly ground black pepper

PLACE THE CHICKEN, CARROTS, CELERY, ONION, GARLIC, SQUASH, BAY LEAF, SALT, AND PEPPER into a large stockpot. Pour in just enough water to cover the chicken and vegetables.

Cover the pot (with the lid tipped a bit) and bring the liquid to a boil over high heat. Reduce the heat to medium low and simmer for about 1½ hours, until the chicken is cooked through and the mixture is very fragrant. Remove the chicken and vegetables from the pot, and pour the liquid through a strainer. On the other side of the strainer should be about 2 quarts of chicken stock. To freeze, place in zip-top storage bags and freeze flat. Defrost easily by running under warm water while still in the bag.

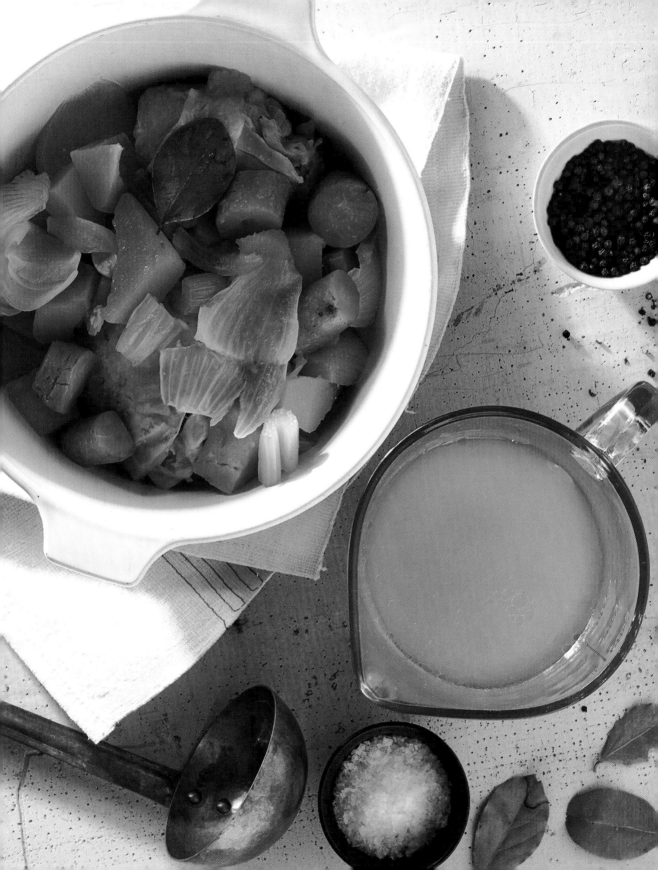

# SCRATCH BLACK BEANS

*Makes* about 6 cups cooked black beans

THESE BEANS ARE WONDERFUL FOR RICE AND BEANS AND CAN EASILY BE TURNED INTO black bean soup or rolled up in tortillas with some cheese and salsa for a quick burrito. They're a shoestring staple. For a vegetarian version of these beans, replace the bacon with 2 to 3 tablespoons of extra-virgin olive oil and 1 teaspoon of kosher salt and proceed with the rest of the recipe as directed. They will still be remarkably flavorful and versatile. This recipe also works well for dried pinto beans, dried black-eyed peas, and dried small red beans (as distinct from kidney beans, which are larger). They all take about the same amount of time to cook using this method.

¼ pound bacon (about 4 to 6 slices), diced

1 large or 2 medium yellow onions, peeled and chopped

6 garlic cloves, peeled and minced

1 pound (16 ounces) dried black beans, rinsed

2 tablespoons balsamic vinegar

2 tablespoons gluten-free soy sauce or tamari

IN A LARGE STOCKPOT, COOK THE BACON OVER MEDIUM-HIGH HEAT, STIRRING OCCASIONALLY, until most of the fat is rendered from it, about 5 minutes. Add the onions to the pot and sauté them in the bacon fat until the onion is translucent, about 6 minutes. Add the garlic and sauté until fragrant, about 2 minutes.

Add the dried black beans to the pot, tossing with the other ingredients to coat. Add 7 to 8 cups of water and simmer, covered, for about 2 hours, or until the beans reach the desired consistency. Check the pot from time to time and add more water if necessary. The beans will absorb more water as they stand after cooking, so you need not be concerned with boiling off the water but rather with softening the beans to the desired tenderness.

Once the beans are cooked to your satisfaction, add the vinegar and tamari or soy sauce, and cook uncovered for 3 to 5 minutes to allow the flavors to come together. Store in a sealed container in the refrigerator for up to 5 days or in the freezer for up to a month. Defrost in the refrigerator.

# DOUGHS
## *and*
# CRUSTS

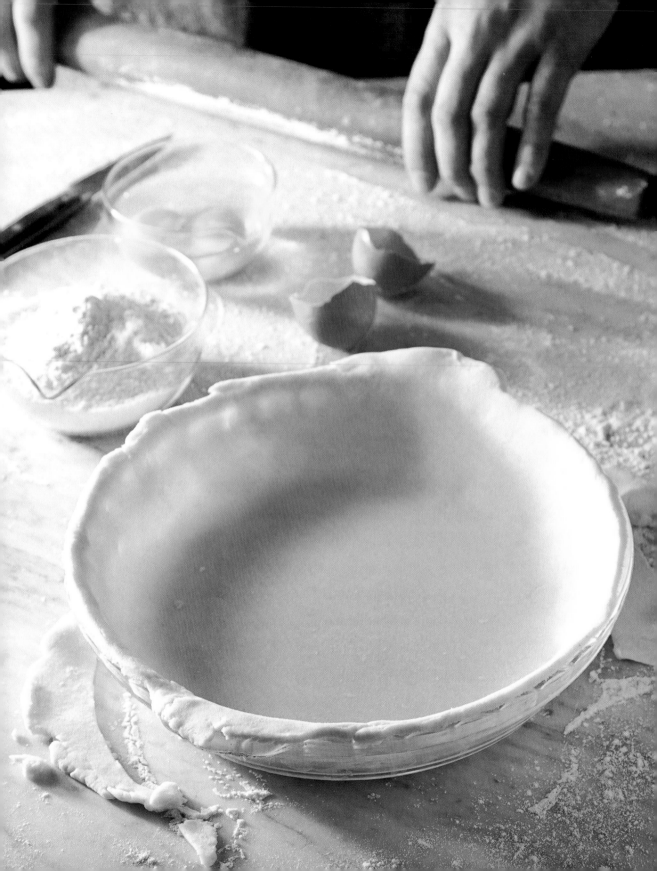

# SWEET PASTRY CRUST

*Makes* enough crust for two 10-inch rounds

THIS RECIPE YIELDS ENOUGH DOUGH TO MAKE THE TOP AND BOTTOM CRUSTS OF A full-size pie. I always make the whole recipe and then freeze whatever I don't need right away, if any. This crust freezes nicely, and it's fabulous for tarts and mini pies, too. In a pinch, it can even be used in place of savory crust (oh, live a little!).

2 cups (280 g) all-purpose gluten-free flour (see page 21)

1 teaspoon xanthan gum (omit if your blend already contains it)

¼ cup (36 g) cornstarch

½ teaspoon (3 g) kosher salt

½ teaspoon baking powder

½ cup (58 g) confectioners' sugar

10 tablespoons (140 g) unsalted butter, chopped and chilled

½ to ¾ cup (4 to 6 fluid ounces) water, iced (ice cubes don't count in the volume measurement)

IN A LARGE BOWL, PLACE THE FLOUR, XANTHAN GUM, CORNSTARCH, SALT, BAKING POWDER, and confectioners' sugar, and whisk until well combined.

Add the cold, chopped butter to the bowl of dry ingredients and toss to coat the butter in the dry ingredients. Using a floured thumb and forefinger or the side of a large spoon, flatten each piece of butter.

Add ½ cup ice water to the mixture by the tablespoon, mixing to combine after each addition, until the dough comes together. Add more water as necessary to moisten any crumbly bits. Divide the dough into two portions, and press each into a disk and wrap separately in plastic. Place in the refrigerator. Chill for at least 30 minutes before rolling out and using as you wish. To freeze the dough for longer storage, wrap tightly in a freezer-safe wrap or container. Defrost in the refrigerator overnight.

*Shoestring* SAVINGS | ON A SHOESTRING: 16¢/ounce
ON THE SHELF: 59¢/ounce

# SAVORY PASTRY CRUST

*Makes* enough crust for two 10-inch rounds

L IKE ITS SWEET COUSIN, THIS RECIPE FOR SAVORY PASTRY CRUST MAKES ENOUGH FOR the top and bottom of a savory pie or quiche. Without baking powder or baking soda, this crust relies only upon the diced butter that expands as the dough bakes, so it's super important that the butter is cold before making the crust and that you use ice water, not just cold tap water. This is one of those basics that will serve you well—and help you breeze through other recipes, like Chicken en Croute (see page 187).

2 cups (280 g) all-purpose gluten-free flour (see page 21)

1 teaspoon xanthan gum (omit if your blend already contains it)

¼ cup (36 g) cornstarch

½ teaspoon (3 g) kosher salt

1 stick plus 2 tablespoons (10 tablespoons) unsalted butter, chopped and chilled

½ to ¾ cup (4 to 6 fluid ounces) water, iced (ice cubes don't count in the volume measurement)

IN A LARGE BOWL, PLACE THE FLOUR, XANTHAN GUM, CORNSTARCH, AND SALT, AND WHISK until well combined.

Add the cold, chopped butter to the bowl of dry ingredients. Using a floured thumb and fore-finger or the side of a large spoon, flatten each piece of butter.

Add ½ cup ice water to the mixture by the tablespoon, mixing to combine after each addition, until the dough comes together. Add more water as necessary to moisten any crumbly bits. Divide the dough into two portions, and press each into a disk and wrap separately in plastic. Place in the refrigerator. Chill for at least 30 minutes before rolling out and using as you wish. To freeze the dough for longer storage, wrap tightly in a freezer-safe wrap or container. Defrost in the refrigera-tor overnight.

# SAVORY OLIVE OIL CRUST

*Makes* enough dough for a top
and bottom crust for one 9-inch pie

I T'S THE OLIVE OIL THAT MAKES THIS CRUST BROWN SO BEAUTIFULLY. OLIVE OIL IS A RICH and flavorful oil, though, so although this crust won't marry well with just any combination of ingredients, it will make a crispy and flaky spinach pie. In fact, it makes a wonderful crust for nearly any quiche.

2 cups (280 g) all-purpose gluten-free flour (see page 21)

1 teaspoon xanthan gum (omit if your blend already contains it)

1 teaspoon (6 g) kosher salt

5 tablespoons (70 g) extra-virgin olive oil

1½ teaspoons white wine vinegar

½ to ¾ cup (4 to 6 fluid ounces) cold water

IN A LARGE BOWL, PLACE THE FLOUR, XANTHAN GUM, AND SALT, AND WHISK TO COMBINE. Pour in the olive oil and vinegar, and stir with a fork to combine. Add ½ cup of cold water and stir until the flour absorbs the water, then mix or knead until the dough comes together. If the dough is crumbly, add more water by the tablespoon, mixing after each addition, until the dough is smooth and pliable.

Cover the dough with plastic wrap, and place it in the refrigerator to chill for 30 minutes or until somewhat firm but not hard. After the dough has chilled, place it between two pieces of unbleached parchment paper, and roll until it is about ⅛ inch thick. Once you have rolled the dough, remove one piece of parchment and dust the dough lightly with extra flour. It is now ready to be used for a savory tart or pie. Simply invert the rolled out crust onto a lightly floured surface, remove the remaining piece of parchment paper, and use as you like.

This dough should not be frozen.

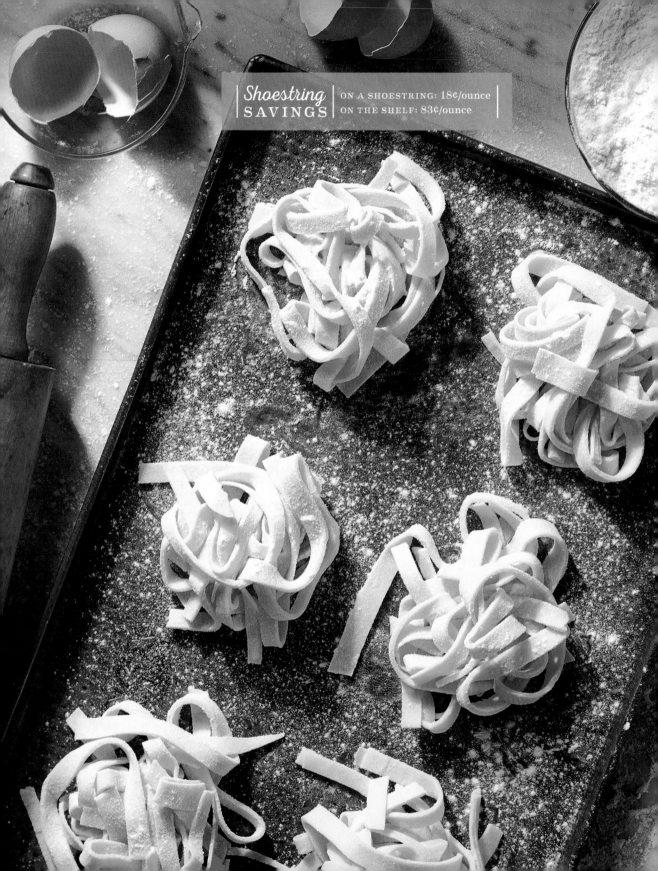

Shoestring
SAVINGS | ON A SHOESTRING: 18¢/ounce
ON THE SHELF: 83¢/ounce

# FRESH PASTA DOUGH

*Makes* enough dough for 12 1½-inch-square ravioli

USE THIS DOUGH TO MAKE RAVIOLI, LASAGNA NOODLES, CANNELLONI, LINGUINI, OR any other shape you like. With so many dried gluten-free pastas readily available at good prices these days, I tend to use this fresh pasta dough for dishes like Spinach and Cheese Ravioli (see page 142), which are less readily available in gluten-free varieties and much, much more expensive. In place of Expandex modified tapioca starch, you can use an equal amount of traditional tapioca starch/flour for similar results. The dough will be a bit more difficult to handle and tear somewhat more easily. Fresh gluten-free pasta is incredibly expensive to buy, with some brands costing $16 for 9 ounces of pasta.

| | |
|---|---|
| 2½ cups plus 3 tablespoons (375 g) all-purpose gluten-free flour (see page 21) | 2 eggs (100 g, weighed out of shell) plus 2 egg yolks (50 g), at room temperature, beaten |
| 1 teaspoon xanthan gum (omit if your blend already contains it) | 1 tablespoon (14 g) extra-virgin olive oil |
| ¼ cup plus 1 tablespoon (45 g) Expandex modified tapioca starch | ¼ cup (2 fluid ounces) warm water, plus more by the ¼ teaspoonful as necessary |
| ½ teaspoon (3 g) kosher salt | |

IN A LARGE BOWL, PLACE THE FLOUR, XANTHAN GUM, EXPANDEX, AND SALT, AND WHISK TO combine well. Create a well in the center of the dry ingredients, add the eggs, egg yolks, olive oil, and ¼ cup warm water and mix to combine. The dough should come together. If there are any crumbly bits, add more remaining warm water by the ¼ teaspoonful until the dough holds together well when squeezed with your hands. Knead together until the dough is smooth and pliable. If it feels stiff, add a few more drops of water and mix in until pliable. It should be, at most, slightly sticky but mostly just smooth.

Transfer the dough to a piece of plastic wrap, wrap it tightly, and allow it to sit at room temperature for about 10 minutes. The dough will absorb more water and any remaining stickiness should dissipate. Unwrap the dough, and divide it in half; return half of it to the plastic wrap, and wrap tightly to prevent it from drying out. Place the remaining half of the dough on a very lightly floured surface, sprinkle very lightly with more flour, and roll into a rectangle about ¼ inch thick.

Flip and shift the dough often to prevent it from sticking, sprinkling only very lightly with more flour as necessary to allow movement. Continue to roll out the dough until it is about ⅛ inch thick. Using a 3-inch round cookie or biscuit cutter, cut out rounds of dough. Remove and gather the trimmings, and reroll them as possible. If you sprinkle the dough with too much flour during shaping, you won't be able to reroll the trimmings. Repeat with the remaining dough.

# PIZZA DOUGH

*Makes* enough crust for two 12-inch pizzas

PIZZA DOUGH IS ONE OF THE SINGLE MOST IMPORTANT STAPLES TO HAVE IN YOUR kitchen. It is exceedingly simple to make, and it even keeps quite well raw in the refrigerator for a few days after you make it. If you make pizza dough at least once every week, then you'll know you can have dinner on the table in less than 30 minutes any night at all. If you'd like to freeze the dough, you must parbake it, which simply means partially baking it, before freezing it. Shape the dough as directed in the recipe, and bake it at 300°F until just set (about 5 minutes). Cool completely, wrap tightly, and freeze for up to 2 months. Before serving, defrost slightly at room temperature, then top and finish baking as directed.

2 cups (280 g) all-purpose gluten-free flour (see page 21)

1½ teaspoons xanthan gum (omit if your blend already contains it)

2 teaspoons (6 g) instant yeast

1 teaspoon (4 g) granulated sugar

1 teaspoon (6 g) kosher salt

3 tablespoons (42 g) extra-virgin olive oil, plus 1 tablespoon for drizzling

¾ cup (6 fluid ounces) warm water (about 90°F)

Toppings, as desired

IN A MEDIUM-SIZE BOWL, THE BOWL OF YOUR FOOD PROCESSOR FITTED WITH THE STEEL blade or stand mixer fitted with the paddle attachment, place the flour, xanthan gum, yeast, and sugar, and whisk to combine with a separate, handheld whisk. Add the salt, and whisk again to combine well.

To the flour mixture, add the 3 tablespoons of olive oil and the water in a steady stream, either pulsing in a food processor, mixing on medium speed in your stand mixer, or mixing with a spoon or fork to combine. If you are using a food processor, pulse while streaming in the water, until a ball begins to form. Otherwise, stir or beat constantly while streaming in the water, and continue stirring until the mixture begins to come together. If the dough seems super sticky, add some more flour, a tablespoon at a time, and stir or pulse to combine. Press the dough into a disk.

Place the dough in another medium-size bowl and drizzle it with olive oil. Turn to coat it with oil. This will prevent a crust from forming on the dough while it is rising. Cover the bowl tightly with plastic wrap and place it in a warm, draft-free area to rise until about 150% its original size (about 1 hour).

After the dough has risen, wrap it in plastic wrap and chill for at least an hour before rolling it out.

To make pizza, roll between two pieces of unbleached parchment paper. Create a crust by rolling the edges thicker, brush the dough with olive oil, and blind bake it at about 400°F (that is, bake it plain, before topping it) for 5 to 7 minutes, so the crust begins to crisp. Then, top it with sauce, cheese, and whatever else you like, and return it to the hot oven until the cheese is melted, about another 5 minutes. Allow to set for 5 minutes before slicing and serving.

*Shoestring* SAVINGS | ON A SHOESTRING: $1.65/crust
ON THE SHELF: $5.00/crust

# WONTON WRAPPERS

*Makes* 15 to 20 wonton wrappers

DID YOU KNOW HOW SIMPLE IT IS TO MAKE YOUR OWN WONTON WRAPPERS? NOT TO worry. That's why you and I are having this talk. And you should feel free to pass it off as your idea. Most likely, you and I don't have any friends in common, so we won't show up at the same gluten-free potluck dinner bearing the very same gluten-free wontons. That would just be embarrassing. In place of Expandex modified tapioca starch, you can use an equal amount of traditional tapioca starch/flour, for similar results. The dough will be a bit more difficult to handle and tear somewhat more easily.

1 ¾ cups (245 g) all-purpose gluten-free flour (see page 21), plus more for sprinkling

¾ teaspoon xanthan gum (omit if your blend already contains it)

35 grams (about ¼ cup) Expandex modified tapioca starch

3 eggs (150 g, weighed out of shell), at room temperature, beaten

¼ to ⅜ cup (2 to 3 fluid ounces) warm water (about 95°F)

IN THE BOWL OF A STAND MIXER FITTED WITH THE PADDLE ATTACHMENT (OR A LARGE BOWL with a wooden spoon), place the flour, xanthan gum, and Expandex, and whisk to combine well with a separate, handheld whisk. Create a well in the center of the dry ingredients, and add the eggs and ¼ cup warm water. Mix to combine on medium speed for about 1 minute (or stir with the wooden spoon for at least 2 minutes). The dough should come together. If there are any crumbly bits, add the remaining warm water by the teaspoon until the dough holds together well when squeezed with your hands. Turn the mixer speed up to medium high, and beat until smooth, 3 to 4 minutes (or by hand with a wooden spoon for at least twice as long). The dough should be smooth and pliable. If it feels stiff, add a few more drops of water and mix in until pliable. It should be, at most, slightly sticky but mostly just smooth.

Transfer the dough to a piece of plastic wrap; wrap it tightly and allow it to sit at room temperature for about 10 minutes. The dough will absorb more water, and any remaining stickiness should dissipate. Unwrap the dough, divide it in half, return half of it to the plastic wrap, and wrap tightly to prevent it from drying out. Place the remaining half of the dough on a lightly floured surface; sprinkle lightly with more flour and roll into a rectangle about ¼ inch thick. Flip and shift the dough often to prevent it from sticking, sprinkling very lightly with more flour as necessary to allow movement. With a pizza wheel, pastry cutter, or sharp knife, trim the edges of the rectangle to create even edges. Remove and gather the trimmings, and set them aside.

Using even and sustained, but not aggressive, pressure, roll out the rectangle until it is approximately ⅛ inch thick. Slice into 3-inch squares. Alternatively, slice the ¼-inch-thick rectangle into 1½-inch squares, and roll each square evenly in all directions until it doubles in surface area and is ⅛ inch thick. I often find this the quicker, easier way to get squares that are the proper thickness.

Use wonton wrappers immediately, or dust any unused wrappers with gluten-free flour and stack. Wrap first in waxed paper and then place in a freezer-safe container; seal tightly and freeze until ready to use. Defrost before using by placing overnight in the refrigerator.

# PÂTE À CHOUX

*Makes* 12 medium-size pastries

PÂTE À CHOUX OR *CHOUX* PASTRY, A LIGHT, SIMPLE BUT SPECIAL FRENCH-STYLE PASTRY dough, looks (and sounds) just beautiful and is just as versatile. With a small switcheroo of a couple ingredients either way, it can be either savory (Gougères, see page 43) or sweet (Profiteroles, see page 43). Made the size of dinner rolls, savory or sweet, they are just right served with an omelet for breakfast or brunch. Super-small *gougères* make delicate cheese puff appetizers. And you only need basic pantry and refrigerator staples, so little to no advance planning is needed to whip up a batch. Beat that with a stick (or a wooden spoon).

1 cup (8 fluid ounces) milk

4 tablespoons (56 g) unsalted butter

½ teaspoon (3 g) kosher salt

1 cup (140 g) all-purpose gluten-free flour (see page 21)

½ teaspoon xanthan gum (omit if your blend already contains it)

4 eggs (200 g, weighed out of shell), at room temperature

Egg wash (1 egg with 1 tablespoon water, beaten)

PLACE THE MILK, BUTTER, AND SALT IN A LARGE SAUCEPAN OVER MEDIUM HEAT UNTIL THE butter is melted and the mixture begins to boil.

Remove the pan from the heat, add the flour and xanthan gum, and stir vigorously. Return to the heat, and continue to stir vigorously for about 3 minutes, until the mixture pulls away from the sides of the pan and comes together in a ball. A thin film will form on the bottom of the pan.

Remove the pan from the heat again, this time for good. Allow the mixture to cool for about 3 to 5 minutes. Line rimmed baking sheets with unbleached parchment paper, and preheat the oven to 425°F.

Add the eggs to the dough, one at a time, stirring the mixture vigorously after each addition. With each egg, the mixture will seem somewhat lumpy. For perfectly smooth dough, place the dough in a food processor fitted with the steel blade, and then add the eggs and pulse until smooth.

Either pipe the dough in mounds through the wide open tip of a pastry bag onto the parchment-lined baking sheets, 2 inches apart from one another, or scoop mounds of dough with a 1½-inch ice-cream scoop onto those same parchment-lined baking sheets, the same 2 inches apart. If you go the pastry bag route, be sure to flatten the tip of each mound with wet fingertips before baking, or it may burn. Brush each puff lightly with the egg wash.

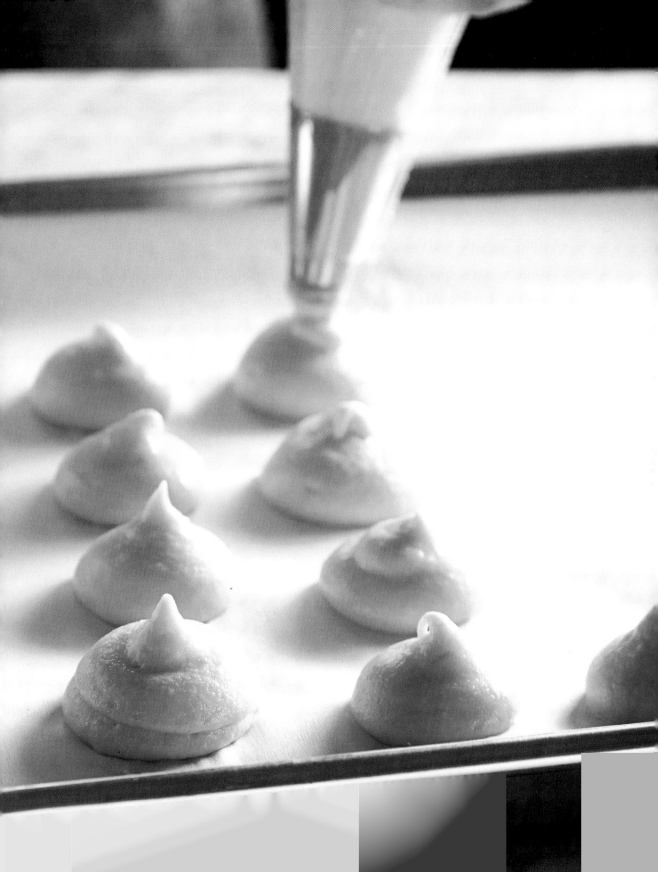

Place baking sheets in the preheated oven and bake 10 minutes at 425°F. Without opening the oven, turn the temperature down to 375°F and finish baking for another 15 to 20 minutes. Five to 10 minutes before the end, open the oven quickly and mark a small X in the top of each puff with a very sharp knife. This will allow steam to escape and help keep the puffs, well, puffy. Continue baking until golden brown.

Allow the puffs to cool at least 5 minutes, 10 if you can stand it. Enjoy with soup, or standing up in the kitchen when no one's looking.

# GOUGÈRES (CHEESE PUFFS)

*Makes* 12 medium-size cheese puffs

To MAKE *GOUGÈRES*, ADD 1 CUP GRATED CHEESE TO THE *PÂTE À CHOUX* DOUGH AFTER adding the eggs to the Pâte à Choux recipe on page 40. You may use any type of grated cheese you like. If authenticity is the name of your game, go with Gruyère cheese. I usually use ⅓ cup Parmesan cheese and ⅔ cup Gruyère (OK, fine, I use ⅔ cup of whatever other grated cheese I have in my refrigerator), but these must be made with dairy cheese. Sadly, nondairy cheese just will not do here.

# PROFITEROLES (CREAM PUFFS)

*Makes* 12 medium-size pastries

To MAKE PROFITEROLES, SUBSTITUTE A PINCH OF SALT FOR THE ½ TEASPOON CALLED for in the Pâte à Choux recipe on page 40 and eliminate the egg wash. After baking, split the little beauties in half horizontally, place vanilla ice cream in the center, and drizzle with melted chocolate mixed with a bit of cream.

# SAUCES
## *and*
# SOUPS

These are your basic sauces. Most use a similar set of
ingredients, and all stay reasonably well in the refrigerator after
being made. The reason is that the acid they contain, typically
in the form of vinegar, keeps them fresh. You make what you
need, in the proportions you like, omitting the ingredients
you don't care for. You will save tons of change, and you will
live a life uncluttered. No longer will your refrigerator door be
littered with bottles of dressings and sauces containing varying
amounts of aging residue. Imagine the clarity you can achieve.
You might very well find yourself writing the next great
American novel. Think of it as kitchen feng shui.

# EASY ENCHILADA SAUCE

*Makes* about 4 cups sauce

I MAKE THIS ENCHILADA SAUCE EVERY SINGLE WEEK. OFTEN, I DOUBLE THE RECIPE AND use half for one meal in a week, the other half for another. I store it in a sealed glass jar in the refrigerator, and it lasts and lasts. It has the perfect balance of spices and can be made with more or less heat, depending upon your family's preferences. I suggest catering to the most heat-sensitive person in your household when making the sauce. Other, more adventuresome members can add more chili powder to their dish, as they like. Spoon this sauce over simple beef tacos, use it to marinate chicken breasts before broiling, baking, or grilling, or use it to make Chicken Enchiladas (see page 193).

6 tablespoons (84 g) unsalted butter, chopped

¼ cup plus 2 tablespoons (54 g) Basic Gum-Free Gluten-Free Flour (see page 21)

1½ cups (12 fluid ounces) Chicken Stock (see page 26)

1 to 2 tablespoons chili powder (depending upon how spicy you like your sauce)

2 teaspoons ground cumin

1 teaspoon smoked Spanish paprika

½ teaspoon garlic powder

1 teaspoon (6 g) kosher salt

1 tablespoon (12 g) granulated sugar

1 (28-ounce) can tomato purée or 1 (28-ounce) can whole, peeled tomatoes in their juice, puréed

1 to 2 tablespoons heavy cream (optional)

IN A MEDIUM, HEAVY-BOTTOM SAUCEPAN, MELT THE BUTTER OVER MEDIUM HEAT. ADD THE flour and whisk until well combined and smooth.

Whisking constantly, slowly add the chicken stock. Continue to cook, whisking frequently, until the mixture begins to bubble and thicken, about 1 minute. Add the chili powder, cumin, paprika, garlic powder, salt, and sugar, and whisk to combine well. Add the tomato purée and whisk, and then stir until well combined.

Add the optional cream to thin as necessary to adjust the heat in the sauce. Serve immediately or cool to room temperature; transfer to a sealed container and store in the refrigerator for up to a week. For longer storage, freeze flat in gallon-size zip-top bags. Defrost by running the frozen bags under warm water before heating and serving.

# CHINESE-STYLE HOT SAUCE

*Makes* about ½ cup sauce

THIS HOT SAUCE IS AN INGREDIENT IN SZECHUAN MEATBALLS (SEE PAGE 172), AND IT also goes nicely with Crispy Asian-Style Tofu (see page 150), Lo Mein (see page 171), and Beef Potstickers (see page 175).

½ teaspoon ground hot red pepper seeds

¼ cup rice vinegar

¼ cup tomato paste

4 teaspoons (28 g) honey

PLACE ALL OF THE INGREDIENTS TOGETHER IN A MEDIUM-SIZE BOWL. WHISK TO COMBINE WELL.

# SWEET AND SOUR SAUCE

*Makes* about ¾ cup sauce

THIS SAUCE PAIRS REALLY WELL WITH CHICKEN, BUT IT'S ALSO DELICIOUS WHEN USED to marinate pork loin or really almost anything fried.

2 tablespoons tamari or gluten-free soy sauce

1 tablespoon (9 g) cornstarch

⅓ cup rice vinegar

¼ cup gluten-free tomato ketchup

¼ cup (50 g) granulated sugar

¾ cup (6 fluid ounces) lukewarm water

IN A MEDIUM-SIZE BOWL, WHISK TOGETHER THE SOY SAUCE, CORNSTARCH, VINEGAR, KETCHUP, and sugar until well combined. Add the water and whisk again to combine.

Pour the mixture into a medium saucepan and cook over medium-high heat, whisking frequently, until it is has thickened and is reduced by about half.

# HOISIN SAUCE

*Makes* about ½ cup sauce

L IKE CHINESE-STYLE HOT SAUCE (SEE PAGE 46), ITSELF AN INGREDIENT IN HOISIN SAUCE, this sauce complements Szechuan Meatballs (see page 172), Crispy Asian-Style Tofu (see page 150), Lo Mein (see page 171), and Beef Potstickers (see page 175).

¼ cup tamari or gluten-free soy sauce

2 tablespoons (32 g) natural peanut butter

1 tablespoon (21 g) honey

2 teaspoons white wine vinegar

⅛ teaspoon garlic powder

2 teaspoons (9 g) toasted sesame oil

⅛ teaspoon freshly ground black pepper

1½ teaspoons Chinese-Style Hot Sauce (optional) (see page 46)

PLACE ALL OF THE INGREDIENTS TOGETHER IN A MEDIUM-SIZE BOWL. WHISK TO COMBINE WELL.

---

# BARBECUE SAUCE

*Makes* about 1 cup sauce

T HIS DELICIOUS BARBECUE SAUCE IS A GREAT PAIRING FOR ANY TRADITIONAL BARBE- cued meat, like roasted chicken parts or ribs, and it also dresses up Meatlove (see page 168) like a champ.

1 cup (8 fluid ounces) gluten-free tomato ketchup

¼ cup (55 g) packed light-brown sugar

2 tablespoons white balsamic or white wine vinegar

1 tablespoon gluten-free Worcestershire sauce

2 teaspoons smoked Spanish paprika

1 teaspoon onion powder

½ teaspoon (3 g) kosher salt

1 tablespoon freshly squeezed lemon juice

IN A SMALL, HEAVY-BOTTOM SAUCEPAN, PLACE ALL OF THE INGREDIENTS AND WHISK TO COMBINE well. Cook, whisking frequently, over medium-low heat until slightly reduced. Remove from the heat and allow to cool to room temperature before serving or storing in the refrigerator in a sealed container.

# EASY HOMEMADE TOMATO SAUCE

*Makes* 7 cups sauce

THIS TOMATO SAUCE IS USED REGULARLY IN MY HOUSE. IT CALLS FOR COOKING BACON, then sautéing onion and garlic in the rendered bacon fat until translucent. Finally, the dried spices, tomato paste, and tomato purée are added. It makes a deeply flavorful sauce in very little time, but it does take about 15 minutes total. When I'm really in a rush and need some tomato sauce to serve with dinner on the double, I simply open a 28-ounce can of good tomato purée (Cento is my favorite brand), add all of the dried spices listed here and the tomato paste, and whisk to combine. I replace the cooked onions and garlic with 1 tablespoon of dried minced onions and ½ teaspoon garlic powder.

¼ pound bacon, diced (optional)

1 to 2 tablespoons (14 to 28 g) extra-virgin olive oil

1 large yellow onion, peeled and grated on a medium-size grater

4 garlic cloves, peeled and grated on a medium-size grater

1 teaspoon (6 g) kosher salt, plus more to taste

½ teaspoon freshly ground black pepper, plus more to taste

1 tablespoon dried basil

2 tablespoons (24 g) granulated sugar

1½ tablespoons dried oregano

1 (6-ounce) can tomato paste

2 (28-ounce) cans tomato purée or 2 (28-ounce) cans whole, peeled tomatoes in their juice, puréed

IF USING BACON, PLACE THE DICED BACON IN A HEAVY-BOTTOM 4-QUART SAUCEPAN AND COOK over medium-high heat, stirring occasionally, until the bacon is crisp-tender (about 4 minutes). Remove the bacon from the pan and set it aside, leaving the rendered bacon fat behind. Add 1 table-spoon of extra-virgin olive oil (2 tablespoons if you did not use bacon), and heat over medium heat until rippling.

Add the grated onions and garlic, and sauté, stirring frequently, until fragrant and beginning to melt (about 4 minutes). Add the salt, pepper, basil, and sugar, and stir to combine. Add the oregano, first rubbing it between your forefinger and palm to release the oils, and stir to combine. Add the tomato paste and tomato purée, and whisk to combine well. Cook until heated through and just beginning to bubble. Add the optional bacon, and stir to combine. Add more salt and/or pepper to taste. Serve hot.

This tomato sauce can be cooled to room temperature and then poured into zip-top freezer bags and frozen flat. That way, it's simple to defrost by running under warm or cool water.

# CREAM OF MUSHROOM SOUP

*Makes* 3½ cups condensed soup

YOU CAN PURCHASE GLUTEN-FREE CREAM OF MUSHROOM SOUP IN A CAN OR IN A shelf-stable box. But, not only is it very expensive, it's just not that flavorful. These recipes for cream of mushroom soup, cream of chicken soup (see page 50), and cream of potato soup (see page 51) can be made up to a week in advance, provided your component ingredients are very fresh. And their flavor can't be beat. Use this cream of mushroom soup to make your famous recipe for green bean casserole around the holidays. It stores quite well in the refrigerator for at least 3 days but tends to separate if frozen.

1 tablespoon (14 g) extra-virgin olive oil

1 small shallot, peeled and minced

1 pound fresh button or baby portabella mushrooms, cleaned and sliced thick

3 tablespoons (42 g) unsalted butter

¼ cup plus 1 tablespoon (45 g) Basic Gum-Free Gluten-Free Flour (see page 21)

¾ teaspoon (almost 5 g) kosher salt

⅛ teaspoon freshly ground black pepper

1½ cups (12 fluid ounces) vegetable stock

1 can (12 fluid ounces) evaporated milk

IN A MEDIUM SAUCEPAN, HEAT THE OLIVE OIL OVER MEDIUM-HIGH HEAT. ADD THE MINCED shallot and mushrooms, and cook until the shallot is translucent and the mushrooms are fork-tender (about 4 minutes). Transfer the mushrooms and shallot to a small bowl and set it aside.

To the same medium saucepan, add the butter and melt over medium heat. Add the flour blend, salt, and pepper, and whisk to combine well. The mixture will clump at first, and then smooth. This is the roux that will thicken the soup. Cook over medium heat, stirring constantly, until the mixture has just begun to turn a very light brown color.

Add the stock to the roux very slowly, whisking constantly to break up any lumps that might form. Add the evaporated milk, and continue to stir until the mixture is smooth. Bring the mixture to a simmer, and continue to cook, stirring occasionally, until reduced by about one-quarter (about 7 minutes). Remove the saucepan from the heat, and add the mushrooms and shallot. Stir to combine.

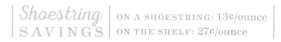

*Shoestring* SAVINGS | ON A SHOESTRING: 13¢/ounce
ON THE SHELF: 27¢/ounce

# CREAM OF CHICKEN SOUP

*Makes* 3½ cups condensed soup

CREAM OF CHICKEN SOUP IS VERY SIMILAR TO CREAM OF MUSHROOM SOUP BUT WITH chicken stock in place of vegetable stock and the addition of chicken and poultry seasoning. To make your own dried poultry seasoning, combine ½ teaspoon dried parsley, 1 teaspoon dried sage, ½ teaspoon dried thyme, ½ teaspoon dried marjoram, and ½ teaspoon rosemary. It's also lovely for adding to Chicken Potpie (see page 181), especially when using store-bought chicken stock, which tends to be less flavorful.

1 tablespoon (14 g) extra-virgin olive oil

1 small shallot, peeled and minced

3 tablespoons (42 g) unsalted butter

¼ cup plus 1 tablespoon (45 g) Basic Gum-Free Gluten-Free Flour (see page 21)

¾ teaspoon (almost 5 g) kosher salt

⅛ teaspoon freshly ground black pepper

1 tablespoon dried poultry seasoning

1½ cups (12 fluid ounces) Chicken Stock (see page 26)

1 can (12 fluid ounces) evaporated milk

1 cup diced cooked chicken

IN A MEDIUM SAUCEPAN, HEAT THE OLIVE OIL OVER MEDIUM-HIGH HEAT. ADD THE MINCED shallot, and cook until translucent (about 4 minutes). Transfer the shallot to a small bowl, and set aside.

To the same medium saucepan, add the butter and melt over medium heat. Add the flour blend, salt, pepper, and poultry seasoning, and whisk to combine well. The mixture will clump at first, and then smooth. This is the roux that will thicken the soup. Cook over medium heat, stirring constantly, until the mixture has just begun to turn a very light brown color.

Add the stock to the roux very slowly, whisking constantly to break up any lumps that might form. Add the evaporated milk, and continue to whisk until the mixture is smooth. Bring the mixture to a simmer, and continue to cook, stirring occasionally, until reduced by about one-quarter (about 7 minutes). Remove the saucepan from the heat, and add the cooked chicken and the shallot. Stir to combine. This condensed soup tends to separate when frozen, and as far as I know, this recipe is not suitable for canning.

# CREAM OF POTATO SOUP

*Makes* 3½ cups condensed soup

CREAM OF POTATO SOUP IS THE MOST ADAPTABLE OF THE THREE CONDENSED SOUP recipes. It can also easily be made into a rich potato soup. Simply increase the amount of peeled and diced potatoes to 1½ pounds. Add more stock to thin to the consistency you prefer, and cook until the potatoes are tender. Finish by puréeing about half the soup with an immersion blender, and garnish with grated cheese and chives.

1 tablespoon (14 g) extra-virgin olive oil

1 small shallot, peeled and minced

3 tablespoons (42 g) unsalted butter

¼ cup plus 1 tablespoon (45 g) Basic Gum-Free Gluten-Free Flour (see page 21)

¾ teaspoon (almost 5 g) kosher salt

⅛ teaspoon freshly ground black pepper

1 teaspoon dry mustard powder (optional)

1½ cups (12 fluid ounces) chicken or vegetable stock

1 can (12 fluid ounces) evaporated milk

½ pound red potatoes, peeled and diced

IN A MEDIUM SAUCEPAN, HEAT THE OLIVE OIL OVER MEDIUM-HIGH HEAT. ADD THE MINCED shallot, and cook until translucent (about 4 minutes). Transfer the shallot to a small bowl, and set aside.

To the same medium saucepan, add the butter and melt over medium heat. Add the flour blend, salt, pepper, and optional mustard powder, and whisk to combine well. The mixture will clump at first, and then smooth. This is the roux that will thicken the soup. Cook over medium heat, whisking constantly, until the mixture has just begun to turn a very light brown color.

Add the stock to the roux very slowly, whisking constantly to break up any lumps that might form. Add the evaporated milk, and continue to whisk until the mixture is smooth. Add the diced potatoes, stir to combine, and bring the mixture to a simmer. Continue to cook, stirring occasionally, until the potatoes are tender and the mixture is reduced by about one-quarter (about 10 minutes). Remove the saucepan from the heat and add the shallot. Stir to combine. This condensed soup tends to separate when frozen, and as far as I know, this recipe is not suitable for canning.

# DIPS
## *and*
# SNACKS

# SPINACH DIP

*Makes* 6 to 8 servings

YOU CAN SERVE THIS FLAVORFUL, CREAMY SPINACH DIP IN A HOLLOWED-OUT BREAD bowl, but there's no way I'd waste a loaf of gluten-free bread by using it as a serving bowl. That would be madness. I just serve it with some chips or sliced raw vegetables.

2 (10-ounce) packages frozen chopped spinach, thawed

½ cup (4 ounces) cream cheese

½ cup (4 ounces) mayonnaise

1 ounce Parmigiano-Reggiano cheese, finely grated

2 ounces low-moisture mozzarella cheese, grated

Juice of 1 large lemon

3 garlic cloves, peeled and minced

1 teaspoon dried parsley flakes

Kosher salt and freshly ground black pepper, to taste

PLACE THE SPINACH IN A FINE MESH BAG OR KITCHEN TOWEL, CINCH THE BAG OR ROLL THE towel closed, and twist to wring out the excess water in the spinach until it wrings dry.

In the bowl of a food processor fitted with the steel blade or a large bowl, place the cream cheese, mayonnaise, Parmigiano-Reggiano and mozzarella cheeses, lemon juice, garlic, parsley, salt, and pepper, and process or mix until smooth. Add the spinach to the mixture and fold it in until the spinach is evenly distributed throughout the dip. Transfer the mixture to a serving bowl and serve chilled or at room temperature.

# TRADITIONAL HUMMUS

*Makes* about 2 cups hummus

THERE ARE MANY BRANDS OF PREPARED HUMMUS THAT ARE RELIABLY GLUTEN-FREE and taste quite good. In my local market, though, they cost nearly four times as much as making hummus at home. The only new ingredient you may have to begin stocking is tahini (sesame paste), which is usually available in conventional supermarkets, on the shelf near the nut butters. A little tahini goes a long way, so you won't need to buy it often.

2 (15-ounce) cans garbanzo beans, drained (not rinsed)

1½ teaspoons (9 g) kosher salt

4 garlic cloves, peeled and minced

⅓ cup tahini (sesame paste)

Juice of 2 lemons

¼ teaspoon lemon zest (optional)

2 to 4 tablespoons (28 to 56 g) extra-virgin olive oil

IN THE BOWL OF A STANDARD-SIZE FOOD PROCESSOR FITTED WITH THE STEEL BLADE, PLACE the garbanzo beans, salt, garlic, tahini, lemon juice, and optional lemon zest. Process until smooth. Add a tablespoon or two of water if necessary to smooth out the texture.

With the food processor switched on, drizzle in 2 tablespoons olive oil. Add up to 2 more tablespoons to taste.

# HOMEMADE JELL-O-STYLE GELATIN

*Makes* 4 servings

MANY IF NOT MOST STORE-BOUGHT DRY GELATIN MIXES ARE SAFELY GLUTEN-FREE. However, if you'd like to make a refined sugar–free, healthy gelatin, this recipe is a real treat. The fruit purée is a really nice touch, but it isn't strictly necessary. You can replace the fruit purée with 1 cup of additional 100 percent fruit juice. You can also replace the honey with 3 to 5 tablespoons (38 to 63 g) granulated sugar, as you like.

1 cup (8 fluid ounces) fruit purée (see instructions below)

1 cup (8 fluid ounces) 100% fruit juice (pineapple or apple juice work well)

1 tablespoon (9 g) unflavored powdered gelatin

2 to 3 tablespoons (42 to 63 g) honey, or to taste

SET ASIDE 4 SINGLE-SERVING HEAT-SAFE DISHES TO HOLD THE GELATIN AS IT SETS.

To make a fruit purée for use in this recipe, soften the fruit by placing it in a heavy-bottom saucepan and adding just enough water to cover it. Bring the mixture to a boil over medium-high heat, stirring occasionally, and cook until pressing it against the side of the pan can easily smash the fruit. For berries, this should only take a couple minutes after boiling. For more fibrous fruits like apples, peel, core, and roughly chop the apples before cooking. It will take longer for the fruit to be tender enough. Once the fruit is ready, remove it from the heat and set it aside to cool for a few minutes before transferring the entire contents of the pan to a blender; purée until smooth. Pass the purée through a fine mesh sieve to remove any solids or seeds. Use only 1 cup (8 fluid ounces) of fruit purée per recipe. If you use more fruit purée than fruit juice, the gelatin will not set up properly.

In a small bowl, place about ¼ cup of the fruit juice and sprinkle with the powdered gelatin. Mix thoroughly and allow to sit until the gelatin swells in the liquid. Place the remaining ¾ cup fruit juice plus 1 cup fruit purée (or more juice) to make 2 full cups in a medium, heavy-bottom saucepan over medium heat. Bring to a boil and remove from the heat. Add the swelled gelatin and honey (or sugar) to the hot saucepan and mix until the honey or sugar and gelatin dissolve.

Immediately divide the mixture among the serving dishes, and allow to cool to room temperature. Cover the dishes and place in the refrigerator to chill until set (about 3 hours) before serving chilled.

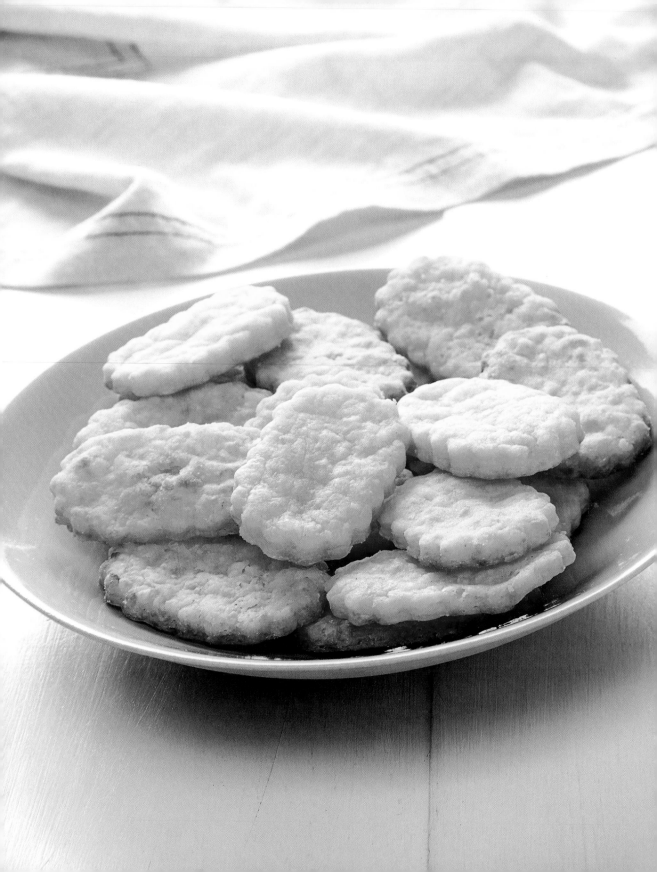

# CHEESE CRACKERS

*Makes* 24 crackers

THESE CRACKERS ARE SUPER SIMPLE, SEDUCTIVELY ELEGANT, INEXPENSIVE TO MAKE, and terribly versatile. As described here, they're rounds. As pictured, they're rectangles. You can make them in any shape you like. Cut the dough into strips, and they're sticks. Roll the strips end over end, and they're sweet little cheese puffs.

| | |
|---|---|
| 1 cup (140 g) all-purpose gluten-free flour (see page 21) | 4 ounces sharp Cheddar cheese, finely grated |
| ½ teaspoon xanthan gum (omit if your blend already contains it) | 6 tablespoons (84 g) unsalted butter, shredded and chilled |
| ¾ teaspoon (about 5 g) kosher salt | ¼ to ⅜ cup (2 to 3 fluid ounces) milk, chilled |

IN A LARGE BOWL, PLACE THE FLOUR, XANTHAN GUM, AND SALT, AND WHISK UNTIL WELL COMbined. Add the cheese and butter, and stir to combine. Add 4 tablespoons of the milk to the mixture, tablespoon by tablespoon, first stirring with a large spoon to combine, then squeezing the mixture with clean, wet hands, adding milk and squeezing until the dough comes together into a cohesive ball. Cover the dough in plastic wrap and place it in the refrigerator until firm, at least 30 minutes.

Once the dough is chilled, preheat the oven to 325°F and line baking sheets with unbleached parchment paper, then set them aside.

Roll out the dough between two sheets of unbleached parchment paper until it's a bit more than ⅛ inch thick (the thickness of a nickel). Uncover the dough by removing the top sheet of parchment, and dust it with more flour. Use a biscuit cutter to cut rounds or other shapes and place them about 1 inch apart on the prepared baking sheets. If the dough has gotten soft at any point, place it in the freezer for a few moments until firm again.

Place in the preheated oven and bake for about 14 minutes, until pale golden brown. Remove from the oven and allow to cool for about 5 minutes on the baking sheet before transferring to a wire rack to cool completely. Store any leftovers in a sealed glass container at room temperature to maintain crispness.

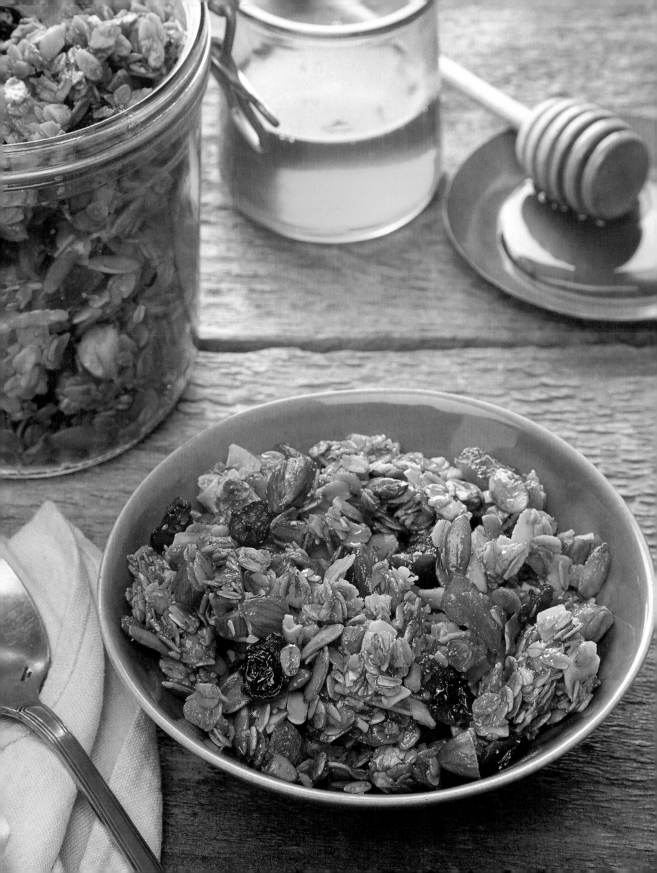

# BREAKFAST *and* BRUNCH, JUST *as* YOU REMEMBER THEM

# TORTILLA ESPAÑOLA

*Makes* 6 to 8 servings (brunch or light dinner),
or many more appetizers

A SPANISH TORTILLA IS NOTHING LIKE THE BREAD-LIKE FLOUR TORTILLAS IN THE chapter on breads (see page 121). It's more like an omelet with onions and potatoes and is often served at room temperature as a light dinner or for brunch. Although I usually dislike using a nonstick pan, as I feel that it's never truly clean even after washing it thoroughly and prefer instead the enameled cast iron of a Dutch oven, a nonstick skillet is essential to making a Tortilla Española. This way you can cook down the sliced potatoes slowly without having them stick to the pan and you can flip the tortilla easily. I have a shallow 10-inch nonstick skillet that I bought largely to be able to make this dish properly. It's also a great pan for shallow frying anything dredged in eggs, like breaded chicken cutlets, and I find it essential for making Arepas (see page 149). Never say never.

4 tablespoons (56 g) extra-virgin olive oil

1 large or 2 medium yellow onions, peeled and chopped

5 to 6 medium potatoes (yellow or red), peeled and sliced ⅛ inch thick

1 tablespoon (18 g) kosher salt

⅛ teaspoon freshly ground black pepper, or to taste

10 eggs (500 g, weighed out of shell)

IN A 10- OR 12-INCH CAST-IRON OR NONSTICK SKILLET, HEAT THE OIL OVER MEDIUM-HIGH heat. Add the onions, and cook for about 6 minutes, until mostly translucent. (If you don't have such a large nonstick skillet, split the recipe in half and use a smaller pan for each half, working in shifts; no big deal.) Add the potatoes, salt, and pepper; cover and cook, stirring occasionally, for about 20 minutes, until the potatoes are wilted and soft.

While the potatoes are cooking away, beat the eggs in a separate bowl, adding just a tiny amount of salt and pepper (the potatoes are already seasoned, remember). When the potatoes are ready, pour the eggs over the top of the potatoes and press them down so they are immersed in the eggs and the top of the mixture is relatively even. Cook over very low heat, covered, about 15 minutes, until the eggs are nearly set. Then remove from the heat and let stand about 5 to 10 minutes covered (until the top is completely set).

It's time to flip the tortilla over to brown the other side. It's much easier than it sounds. First, gently shake the skillet to make sure that the tortilla is not stuck to the bottom of the pan. If it does seem a bit stuck, run a heatproof spatula along the edge of the tortilla to free it. Now place a large plate firmly on top of the skillet and, stepping lively, invert the plate and skillet together.

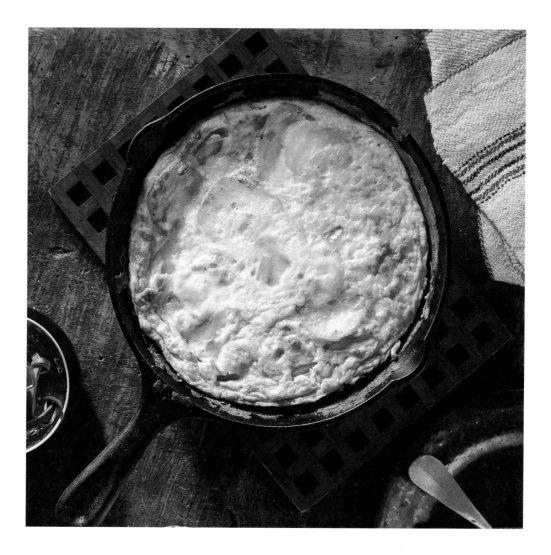

Remove the skillet from the top. Now simply slide the tortilla from the plate back into the skillet, shimmying the plate as you go.

Cover and cook again over very low heat for about 5 minutes. Slide off the skillet and onto a plate and serve either warm or at room temperature. There are a few traditional Spanish ways to serve it: for tapas, cut it into squares with toothpicks inserted into each square, or separate off a rectangle of the tortilla and serve it on a roll.

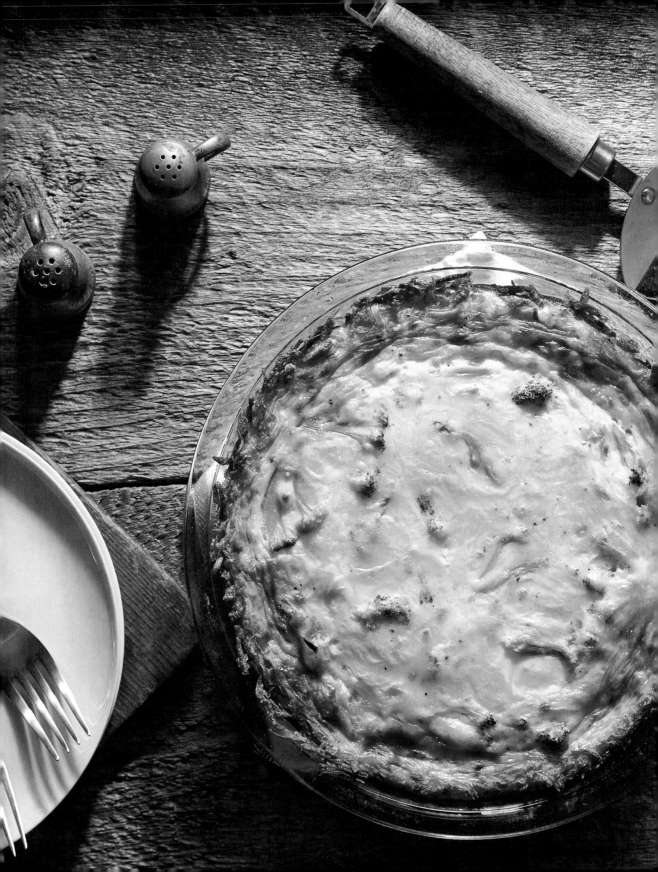

# OVEN HASH BROWN QUICHE

*Makes* 4 to 6 servings

I OFTEN MAKE OVEN HASH BROWNS. I JUST PEEL AND GRATE POTATOES, WRING THEM DRY, and then toss them with kosher salt, pepper, and canola oil and bake them in a rimmed baking sheet in one layer in a 400°F oven for 15 to 20 minutes. Then I cut the hash browns into squares with kitchen shears and serve topped with scrambled eggs. It's super tasty, easy, inexpensive, and even looks elegant. This quiche starts with the same principle but uses the oven hash browns as a crust for a quiche. Crispy on the underside and creamy toward the middle, it makes a lovely brunch.

4 medium potatoes (yellow or red), peeled and grated

½ teaspoon (3 g) kosher salt

⅛ teaspoon freshly ground black pepper

3 to 4 tablespoons (42 to 56 g) vegetable oil

8 ounces frozen broccoli florets

8 eggs (400 g, weighed out of shell), at room temperature, beaten

1 can (12 fluid ounces) evaporated milk

4 ounces Cheddar or mozzarella cheese, grated

4 ounces Parmigiano-Reggiano cheese, finely grated

PREHEAT THE OVEN TO 375°F. GREASE A 9-INCH GLASS PIE PLATE WITH UNSALTED BUTTER AND set it aside.

Place the grated potatoes in a kitchen towel or fine mesh bag and wring to squeeze out as much water from the potatoes as possible. Place them in a large bowl. Toss the potatoes with the salt, pepper, and oil. Press the potatoes evenly into the bottom and sides of the prepared pie plate. Place the pie plate into the center of the preheated oven and bake for 10 to 15 minutes, or until the potatoes are just beginning to brown on top and around the bottom. You're using a glass pie plate so you can sneak a look at the crust as it browns.

While the hash brown crust is browning, defrost and drain the broccoli, then chop it into bite-size pieces. In a large bowl, whisk together the eggs and milk. Stir in the grated cheese and broccoli.

Remove the hash brown crust from the oven and pour the egg mixture into the center of the pie plate. Place the quiche in the center of the oven and bake for about 35 to 45 minutes, or until the eggs are set and golden around the edges, and you can see by looking through the bottom of the pie plate that the crust has browned nicely.

Allow to set for 5 to 10 minutes. Slice into wedges and serve.

# RICOTTA PANCAKES

*Makes* 4 servings

Ricotta pancakes have comparatively little flour compared to traditional pancakes and a touch more sugar. The moisture from the ricotta cheese keeps the pancakes so moist that they're almost custard-like toward the center. They're also rich and creamy and just a bit more special than your everyday pancake.

⅔ cup (93 g) Basic Gum-Free Gluten-Free Flour (see page 21)

¼ cup (50 g) sugar

½ teaspoon (3 g) kosher salt

1 teaspoon baking powder

2 eggs (100 g, weighed out of shell), at room temperature, beaten

1 cup (250 g) low-moisture ricotta cheese, at room temperature

½ cup (4 fluid ounces) milk, at room temperature

2 teaspoons pure vanilla extract

In a large bowl, place the flour, sugar, salt, and baking powder, and whisk to combine. In a separate small bowl, place the eggs, ricotta cheese, milk, and vanilla extract, and beat to combine well. Create a well in the center of the dry ingredients, add wet ingredients, and beat until smooth. The batter should be thick but pourable.

Heat a griddle or greased nonstick or cast-iron skillet over medium heat. Grease it lightly, and pour as many portions of about ¼ cup of batter onto the hot griddle as can fit comfortably without touching.

Allow to cook until large bubbles begin to break through the top of the batter in each pancake and the edges are set (about 2 minutes). With a wide, flat spatula, carefully flip over each pancake, and continue to cook just until set (about another minute). Remove from the skillet, and repeat with the remaining batter. Serve immediately.

These pancakes can be cooled, stacked, wrapped very tightly, and then frozen for at least a month. Defrost by placing in a toaster oven or standard oven at a very low temperature until warmed through.

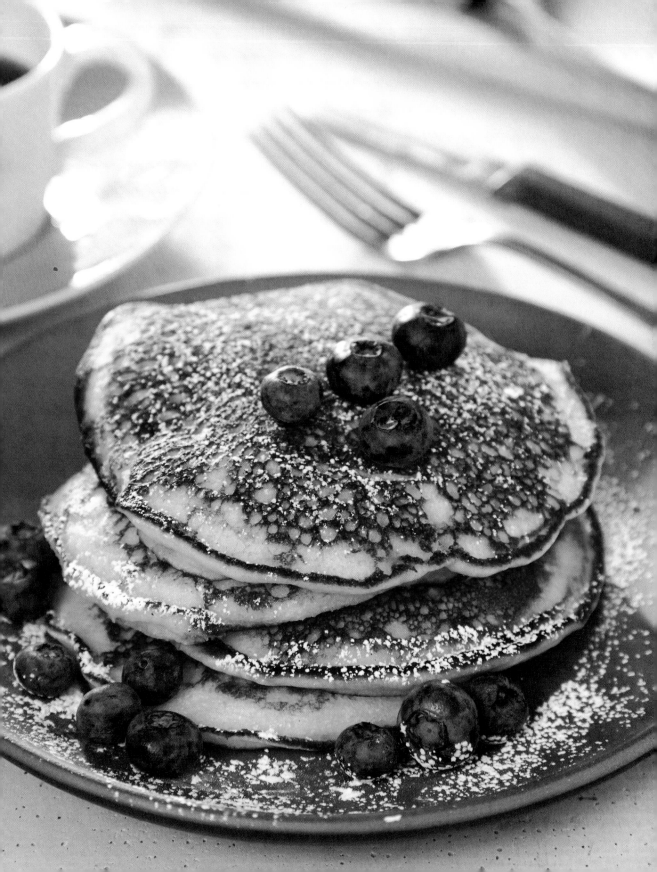

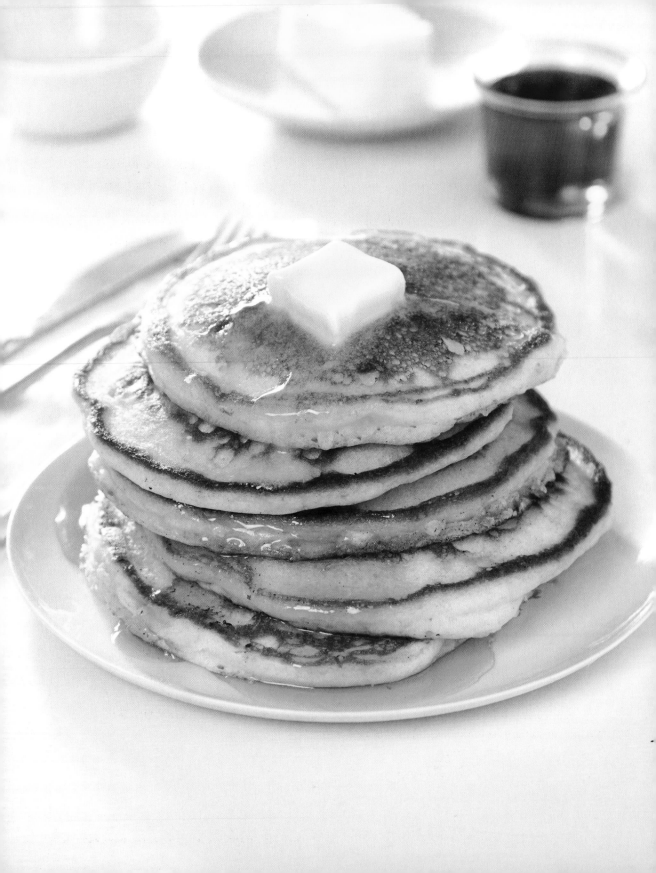

# BUTTERMILK PANCAKES

*Makes* 4 servings

LIGHT AND FLUFFY BUTTERMILK PANCAKES ARE YOUR EVERYDAY PANCAKES. THE BUTTER-milk gives them that creamy richness and slight tang, and the bit of sugar some sweetness. You can leave out the sugar entirely if you prefer. For an extra-special, no-mess maple syrup experience, try drizzling some cold maple syrup in a swirl on the raw side of a just-poured pancake. The syrup will seep into the batter as it sets, flavoring the whole pancake. Cold syrup is thicker, so it will pour more slowly, giving you more control as you swirl.

1¼ cups (175 g) Basic Gum-Free Gluten-Free Flour (see page 21)

¼ teaspoon xanthan gum (optional—will keep the edges of the pancakes from feathering)

1½ teaspoons baking powder

½ teaspoon baking soda

½ teaspoon (3 g) kosher salt

2 tablespoons (24 g) granulated sugar

2 eggs (100 g, weighed out of shell), at room temperature, beaten

¾ cup (6 fluid ounces) buttermilk, at room temperature

2 tablespoons (28 g) unsalted butter, melted and cooled

IN A LARGE BOWL, PLACE THE FLOUR, OPTIONAL XANTHAN GUM, BAKING POWDER, BAKING soda, salt, and sugar, and whisk to combine well. Set the bowl aside. In a large, spouted measuring cup, place the eggs, buttermilk, and butter, and whisk vigorously to combine well and beat the eggs completely. Create a well in the center of the dry ingredients and add the buttermilk and egg mixture in a slow, steady stream, whisking constantly. Continue to whisk until the mixture is smooth. It will be thick.

Heat a griddle or greased nonstick or cast-iron skillet over medium heat. Grease it lightly, and pour as many portions of about ¼ cup of batter onto the hot griddle as can fit comfortably without touching. When pouring the batter, don't swirl it around; pour straight down.

For extra-thick pancakes, allow the pancakes to cook until the edges are beginning to set, and then add more batter right to the center of the pancake. Allow the pancakes to cook until large bubbles begin to break through the top of the batter in each pancake and the edges are set (about 2 minutes). With a wide, flat spatula, carefully flip over each pancake, and continue to cook until set (about another minute). Remove from the skillet, and repeat with the remaining batter.

Pancakes can be cooled completely and then stacked, wrapped tightly, and frozen. Separate the pancakes and defrost in the toaster oven on light or low.

*Shoestring* SAVINGS | ON A SHOESTRING: 20¢/each
ON THE SHELF: $1.15/each

# BANANA PANCAKE MUFFINS

*Makes* 12 pancake muffins

THESE LIGHT AND FLUFFY LITTLE PANCAKE MUFFINS ARE BAKED IN THE OVEN UNTIL they're a pale golden brown. You can serve them nearly straight from the oven or even refrigerate and reheat them the next day. They don't taste like traditional muffins, since the batter is nearly the same as pancakes cooked on a griddle or in a pan. They taste like, well, banana pancakes, but you can hold them in your hand, and everyone can eat together since they're all ready at the same time.

2 cups (280 g) all-purpose gluten-free flour (see page 21)

1 teaspoon xanthan gum (omit if your blend already contains it)

½ teaspoon baking soda

1 teaspoon baking powder

1 teaspoon (6 g) kosher salt

2 tablespoons (24 g) granulated sugar

1 egg (50 g, weighed out of shell), at room temperature, lightly beaten

1½ cups (12 fluid ounces) milk

1½ teaspoons white wine vinegar

2 tablespoons (28 g) unsalted butter, melted and cooled

2 ripe bananas (200 g), diced

PREHEAT THE OVEN TO 375°F. GREASE OR LINE THE WELLS OF A STANDARD 12-CUP MUFFIN TIN and set it aside.

In a large bowl, place the flour, xanthan gum, baking soda, baking powder, salt, and sugar, and whisk to combine. Add the egg, milk, vinegar, and butter, mixing to combine after each addition. Add the diced bananas to the batter, and fold gently until they are evenly distributed throughout.

Divide the pancake batter among the wells of the muffin tin and bake for about 20 minutes or just until they are not wet in the middle. Cool for 5 minutes in the muffin tin, then serve when still warm.

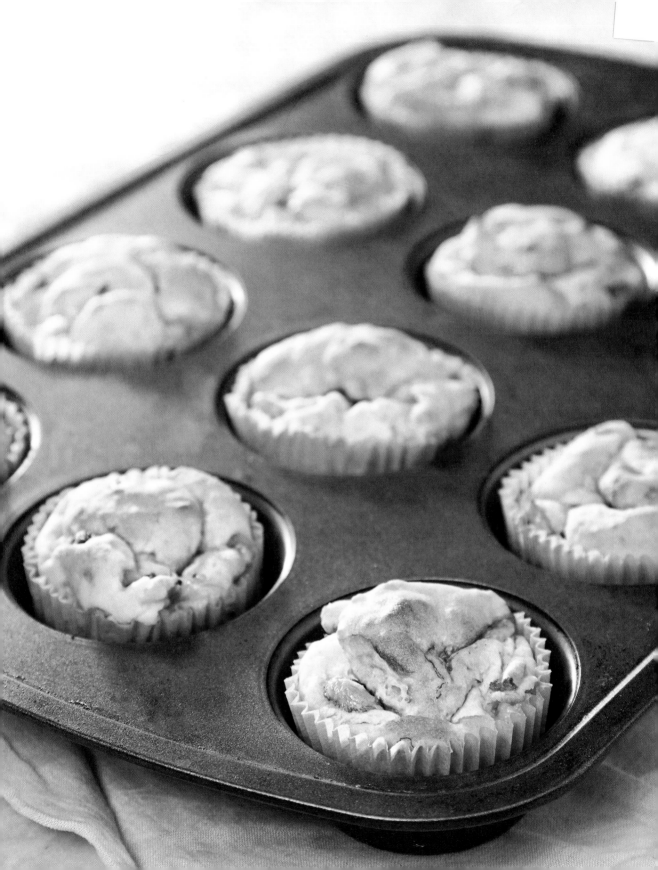

# SOFT AND FLUFFY WAFFLES

*Makes* 8 square or 4 Belgian waffles

WAFFLES ARE SORT OF LIKE PANCAKES WITH WINGS. THEIR DELICATE, CRISP-fluffiness comes from separating the eggs and whipping the whites separately. You just have to lean into it. Be sure not to overbeat the egg whites or they'll appear to crumble a bit. It's important that you use oil, not butter, as oil has essentially no water in it. The water in butter will make it much more likely for the waffle batter to melt over the sides of the waffle iron as it heats.

2 cups (280 g) Gum-Free Gluten-Free Flour (see page 21)

2 tablespoons (24 g) sugar

1½ teaspoons baking powder

½ teaspoon baking soda

½ teaspoon (3 g) kosher salt

2 eggs (100 g, out of shell), at room temperature, separated

3 tablespoons (42 g) virgin coconut oil, melted and cooled, or neutral oil (vegetable or canola)

1 cup (227 grams) plain whole milk yogurt

¾ cup (6 fluid ounces) milk, at room temperature

PREHEAT AND PREPARE YOUR WAFFLE IRON ACCORDING TO THE MANUFACTURER'S DIRECTIONS. In a large bowl, place the flour blend, xanthan gum, sugar, baking powder, baking soda, and salt, and whisk to combine well. In a separate bowl, whip the egg whites with a hand mixer (or in a stand mixer fitted with the whisk attachment) until stiff (but not dry) peaks form. Place the egg yolks and oil in a separate large bowl and blend with a hand mixer (or in a stand mixer fitted with the paddle attachment) until creamy. Add the yogurt and milk, and blend until well combined. Add the dry ingredients, and blend again. The mixture will be smooth and thick but pourable. Fold the beaten egg whites gently into the large bowl of batter until only a few white streaks remain.

Pour or scoop about ¾ to 1 cup of batter into your prepared waffle iron (more or less depending upon the size and shape of your iron), and spread the batter into an even layer. Close the lid and cook until steam stops escaping from the waffle iron, between 4 and 5 minutes, depending again upon the capacity of your waffle iron. Remove the waffle from the iron and serve immediately. Repeat with the remaining batter.

If you do not serve each waffle as soon as it is made, refresh the waffles by placing them in a toaster oven at 400°F for about 3 minutes. Waffles can also be cooled completely, wrapped tightly, and frozen, and then defrosted and refreshed in a similar manner before serving.

# EASY OATMEAL
# BREAKFAST COOKIES

*Makes* 10 generous breakfast cookies

THESE ARE DAIRY-FREE AND LOW IN FAT BUT RICH IN WHOLE GRAINS. THE CHOCOLATE chips or raisins are a nice touch but not entirely necessary. I like to use miniature chocolate chips when I'm trying to get away with using less chocolate. They scatter and cover more ground in a cookie. You can easily grind your own oat flour from oats in a blender or food processor.

1¼ cups (125 g) certified gluten-free old-fashioned rolled oats

1½ cups (180 g) certified gluten-free oat flour

½ teaspoon baking soda

½ teaspoon kosher salt

5 tablespoons (70 g) virgin coconut oil, melted and cooled

5 tablespoons (105 g) honey

½ cup (122 g) smooth applesauce, at room temperature

2 eggs (100 g, weighed out of shell), at room temperature, beaten

3 ounces miniature chocolate chips or raisins

PREHEAT THE OVEN TO 350°F. LINE A RIMMED BAKING SHEET WITH UNBLEACHED PARCHMENT paper and set aside.

In a large bowl, place the oats, oat flour, baking soda, and salt, and mix to combine. Add the oil, honey, applesauce, and eggs, and mix to combine. The dough will be very soft. Add the chips or raisins to the mix until evenly distributed throughout. Refrigerate or freeze the dough briefly to make it easier to handle before dividing it into 10 equal portions and placing on the prepared baking sheet, about 1½ inches apart from one another. A medium ice-cream scoop works quite well to portion the dough. Chill until firm (about 10 minutes). This keeps the cookies from spreading too much during baking.

Place in the preheated oven, and bake until golden brown around the edges and set in center (about 16 minutes). Cool on the baking sheet until firm before serving. Wrap any leftovers in waxed paper and store in the refrigerator or freezer.

# APPLE-CINNAMON
# TOASTER PASTRIES

*Makes* 12 toaster pastries

WHEN I WAS KID, BROWN SUGAR AND CINNAMON POP-TARTS TOASTER PASTRIES were my breakfast of champions. Knowing now what was in them (in a word: sugar), it's no wonder I was hungry again in an hour. These Apple-Cinnamon Toaster Pastries have real ingredients, including a substantial apple filling. But they're still a treat. If only I could pretend that they were healthy enough to eat for breakfast every day, I'd surely join my children every single morning for a lightly toasted pastry, with the perfect shortbread-style crust, filled with apple-cinnamon goodness.

PASTRY

2 ¼ cups (315 g) all-purpose gluten-free flour (see page 21)

1 teaspoon xanthan gum (omit if your blend already contains it)

¼ cup (36 g) cornstarch

½ teaspoon (3 g) kosher salt

¾ cup (150 g) granulated sugar

8 tablespoons (112 g) unsalted butter, melted and cooled

1 teaspoon pure vanilla extract

1 egg (50 g, weighed out of shell), at room temperature, beaten

¼ to ⅜ cup (2 to 3 fluid ounces) milk, at room temperature

FILLING

4 firm apples, peeled, cored, and grated

1 teaspoon pure vanilla extract

¼ teaspoon (about 1 g) kosher salt

1 teaspoon ground cinnamon

½ cup (109 g) packed light-brown sugar

2 teaspoons (6 g) cornstarch

PREHEAT THE OVEN TO 350°F. LINE BAKING SHEETS WITH UNBLEACHED PARCHMENT PAPER and set aside.

In a large bowl, place the flour, xanthan gum, cornstarch, salt, and sugar, and whisk to combine well. Create a well in the center of the dry ingredients and add the butter, vanilla, egg, and ¼ cup of the milk, mixing to combine after each addition. The dough will be thick. Knead the dough with your hands until it is smooth, adding more milk by the ½ teaspoonful as necessary to bring the dough together. Place the dough on a lightly floured surface and dust lightly with flour to prevent it from sticking. Roll out the dough ¼ inch thick and slice it into 4 ½ × 3 ½-inch rectangles. Gather and reroll any scraps, and cut out as many more rectangles as possible. You should have at least 24 rectangles.

Prepare the filling. In a medium saucepan, place the apples, vanilla, salt, and cinnamon, plus ¼ cup (2 fluid ounces) water, and stir to combine. Cook over medium-high heat for about 5 minutes, stirring frequently, until the apples are very soft. Once the apple mixture is cooked, remove the saucepan from the heat. Add the brown sugar and cornstarch, and stir until they dissolve, with no lumps.

Place 12 of the pastry rectangles on the prepared baking sheet, about 1 inch apart. Divide the filling evenly among the rectangles, spreading out the filling but leaving a border of about ½ inch from the edges. Place the remaining 12 pastry rectangles atop the 12 with filling and press down the edges of the pastry to seal them. Trim the edges slightly using a pastry wheel or sharp knife. Pierce the tops of the pastries randomly with a toothpick to allow steam to escape during baking.

Place the baking sheet in the center of the preheated oven and bake for about 10 minutes, or until the pastries are very lightly golden brown and just set in the center. Serve immediately, or allow to cool completely and wrap tightly and freeze until ready to serve. Defrost in the toaster oven on a very light setting or very low heat until just warmed.

*Shoestring* SAVINGS | ON A SHOESTRING: 50¢/each
ON THE SHELF: $1.20/each

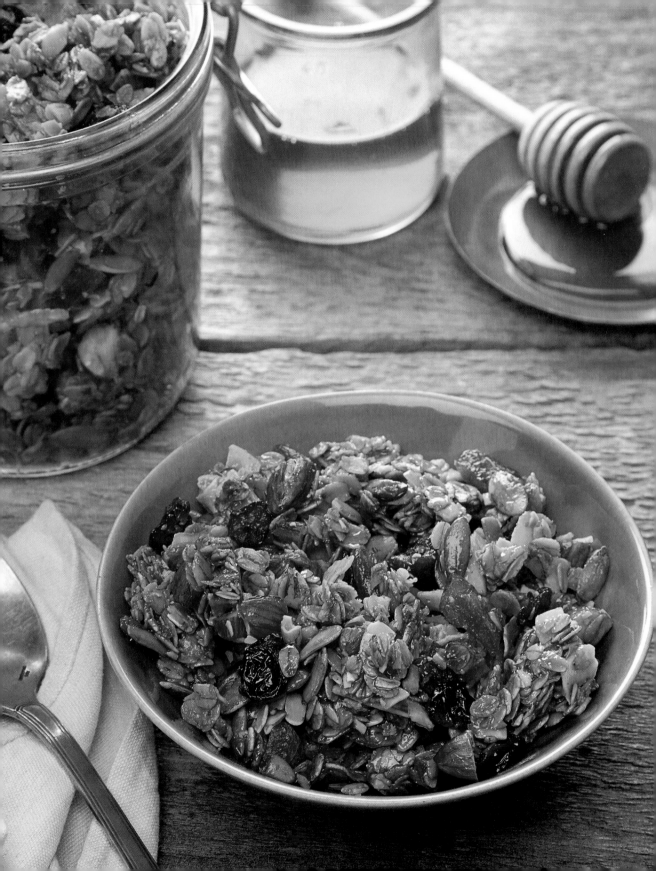

# HOMEMADE CRUNCHY GRANOLA

*Makes* about 5 cups granola

EVEN CONVENTIONAL GRANOLA IS ONE OF THOSE FOODS THAT CAN COST YOU A KING'S ransom, but it seems that no one knows why that is. And don't get me started on the cost of gluten-free granola. Take heart, though, dear friends: you can create your own home-made, gluten-free granola, modified to your particular tastes, whichever way they run, and have it all done before you can say "Bob's your uncle." The almonds and the oats are somewhat compulsory, or it's not really granola, and you'll certainly need some honey and some oil. But the dried fruit you choose is your business. Just be sure to add it to the granola after it's finished baking to prevent the fruit from hardening in the oven.

4 tablespoons (56 g) neutral oil

½ cup (168 g) honey

½ teaspoon (3 g) kosher salt

3 cups (300 g) certified gluten-free old-fashioned rolled oats

1 cup (120 g) sliced almonds

½ cup (75 g) dried cranberries (preferably unsweetened)

½ cup (75 g) raisins (I like Thompson seedless raisins)

PREHEAT THE OVEN TO 300°F. LINE A LARGE RIMMED BAKING SHEET WITH UNBLEACHED parchment paper and set it aside.

In a small saucepan over low heat, heat the oil, honey, and salt, stirring occasionally, until the honey has melted and the mixture is warmed throughout (3 to 5 minutes).

While the honey and oil are warming, in a separate large bowl, add the oats and almonds, and stir until well combined. When the honey mixture is ready, pour it over the oat mixture and stir with a wet spatula (to prevent the honey from clumping) until the honey mixture has coated the oat mixture completely. Scrape the mixture onto the prepared baking sheet and spread it out in a single, even layer.

Place the baking sheet in the center of the preheated oven and bake for 15 minutes. Remove the baking sheet from the oven, stir it to redistribute, and return it to the oven. Bake for another 10 minutes, stir once more, and continue baking until lightly golden brown all over (about 10 minutes more). Remove it from the oven, add the dried fruit, and stir gently to distribute it evenly throughout the granola. Allow the granola to cool completely on the baking sheet. Break it up into irregular chunks and serve. It can be stored in a sealed glass container at room temperature for at least 2 weeks.

*Shoestring* SAVINGS | ON A SHOESTRING: $1.39/cup
ON THE SHELF: $2.54/cup

BREAKFAST AND BRUNCH, JUST AS YOU REMEMBER THEM

# PLAIN BAGELS

## *Makes* 8 bagels

M Y SON CAME HOME ONE DAY AND ANNOUNCED, NICE AS YOU PLEASE, THAT TOMOR-
row he would be needing a green bagel for a St. Patrick's Day celebration in school—
where of course, everyone else would be eating a gluten-filled green bagel. The moral
of the story is this: you never know when such an announcement might be made in your house.
(And if it is, a few drops of plain, water-based McCormick green food color in the warm water
called for in the recipe below is all you need.) So you've got to be prepared. It is with these sorts of
adventures in mind that I present the following basic recipe for a chewy-on-the-outside, fluffy-
on-the-inside bagel.

The recipe in the first edition of this cookbook for plain bagels was made in the "old" gluten-
free bread style, using an all-purpose gluten-free flour. At the time, it seemed like a revolution!
Since then, I've raised the bar for gluten-free bread. This recipe is in that new style.

3½ cups (490 g) Gluten-Free Bread
Flour (see page 21), plus more for
sprinkling

2 teaspoons (6 g) instant yeast

2 tablespoons (24 g) granulated sugar

1½ teaspoons (9 g) kosher salt

1 cup plus 1 tablespoon (8½ fluid
ounces) warm water (about 95°F)

6 tablespoons (84 g) unsalted butter,
at room temperature

Bath for boiling (6 cups water plus
1 tablespoon molasses plus
1 teaspoon salt)

Egg wash (1 egg plus 1 tablespoon
milk, beaten)

PREHEAT THE OVEN TO 400°F. LINE A LARGE RIMMED BAKING SHEET WITH UNBLEACHED
parchment paper, spray it with nonstick cooking spray, and set it aside.

In the bowl of your stand mixer (or a large bowl with a handheld mixer with dough hooks),
place the bread flour, yeast, and granulated sugar, and use a handheld whisk to combine well.
Add the salt and whisk to combine well. Add the warm water and butter, and mix on low speed
with the dough hook(s) until combined. Raise the mixer speed to medium and knead for about 5
minutes. The enriched dough will be smooth and very thick. Spray a silicone spatula lightly with
cooking oil spray, and scrape down the sides of the bowl. Cover the bowl with plastic wrap and
place in the refrigerator to chill for 10 minutes to make the dough easier to handle.

Remove the dough from the refrigerator, and transfer it to a surface lightly sprinkled with
bread flour. Sprinkle the dough very lightly with more flour and turn it over on itself a few times
until the dough is smoother. Using a bench scraper or sharp knife, divide the dough into 8 equal
pieces. Working with one piece of dough at a time on a well-floured surface, flatten the dough

into a disk. Pull the edges toward the center of the disk and secure the edges together by pressing them between your thumb and forefinger. Turn the dough over so that the gathered edges are on the bottom and cup your whole hands around the dough to coax it into a round shape. Place the round of dough on a lightly floured surface and cup only one palm around the dough with the side of your hand resting on the counter (the side of your hand nearest your pinkie). Maintaining contact between the side of your hand and the surface, begin to move your hand in a circular motion while gently coaxing the edges of the dough upward (toward the top of the round) with the tips of your fingers.

Place each round of dough about 2 inches apart from one another on the prepared baking sheet after shaping. Place a floured finger in the center of each round of dough, press down to the bottom and move around in a circular motion to create a hole that is at least 1½ inches wide.

Place the ingredients of the molasses bath in a medium saucepan, and bring to a boil over medium-high heat. Place as many of the raw, shaped bagels in the boiling water bath as can fit without crowding, and boil them for about 45 seconds total, turning the bagels over gently to ensure even boiling. Remove the boiled bagels from the bath and return to the baking sheet. Brush the tops and sides with the egg wash.

Place the baking sheet in the center of the preheated oven and bake until the bagels are golden brown all over and the internal temperature reaches about 180°F (18 to 20 minutes). Remove from the oven and allow to cool briefly before serving.

These freeze quite well. Simply cool completely, and then slice in half through the center (as one does with a bagel). Wrap very tightly in a freezer-safe bag, squeezing out all the air, and freeze for up to a month. Defrost in a toaster oven on the lowest setting.

# CINNAMON ROLLS

*Makes* 12 cinnamon rolls

AFTER SANDWICH BREAD (SEE PAGE 109), CINNAMON ROLLS WERE ONE OF THE VERY first yeast bread recipes I ever developed when I started baking gluten-free. Warm, gooey, swirled rolls filled with cinnamon and sugar are practically a food group. Being able to make them gluten-free was an obvious necessity early on. They take a bit of time to shape, rise, and bake, but they're worth it on holiday mornings or for a special Sunday brunch.

This recipe for yeasted cinnamon rolls is in the original style of gluten-free bread baking, just as it appeared in the first edition of this book. We're going old school this time.

DOUGH

6 tablespoons (84 g) unsalted butter, melted and cooled to room temperature

¼ cup (50 g) granulated sugar

2 eggs (100 g, weighed out of shell) plus 3 egg yolks (75 g), at room temperature

½ teaspoon (3 g) kosher salt

1½ cups (12 fluid ounces) buttermilk, at room temperature

3 cups (420 g) all-purpose gluten-free flour (see page 21)

2 teaspoons xanthan gum (omit if your blend already contains it)

2 teaspoons (6 g) instant yeast

FILLING

¾ cup (164 g) packed light-brown sugar

2 tablespoons (28 g) unsalted butter, melted and cooled

2 teaspoons ground cinnamon

⅛ teaspoon (almost 1 g) kosher salt

IN THE BOWL OF A STAND MIXER FITTED WITH THE PADDLE ATTACHMENT OR A LARGE BOWL with a spoon, place the butter, sugar, eggs, egg yolks, and salt, and mix to combine well. Add the buttermilk, and mix until smooth. To the wet ingredients, add the flour, xanthan gum, and yeast, beating well after each addition. The dough will be sticky, but you should be able to handle it with some maneuvering. If it seems super sticky, add more flour a tablespoon at a time and beat or stir to combine.

Grease a 13 × 9-inch baking dish with unsalted butter and set it aside. To make the filling, in a medium bowl, place the brown sugar, butter, cinnamon, and salt, and mix with a fork until a paste forms. Set the bowl aside.

Place the dough between two sheets of unbleached parchment paper. Roll the dough into a square that is approximately 12 by 12 inches. Remove the top sheet of parchment. Spread the filling mixture onto the exposed dough, gently so as to avoid tearing the dough, leaving a 1-inch clean border all around. Moisten the bare 1-inch border with wet fingers. Beginning with one side of the dough and using the parchment to coax the dough neatly, roll the dough into a cylinder as tightly as possible, pinch the seam to seal it well, and place it on the flat surface seam-side down. Using a sharp knife or a piece of unwaxed dental floss, slice the cylinder into 12 cross-sections, each about 1 inch thick. Arrange the cinnamon rolls about 1 inch apart in the prepared baking dish.

Cover the baking dish tightly with plastic wrap and place it in a warm, draft-free area to rise until the rolls are about 150 percent of their original volume (about 1 hour). When the dough is nearing the end of its rise, preheat the oven to 350°F.

Remove the plastic wrap from the baking dish, and place it in the center of the preheated oven and bake for about 30 minutes, or until golden brown. Serve immediately.

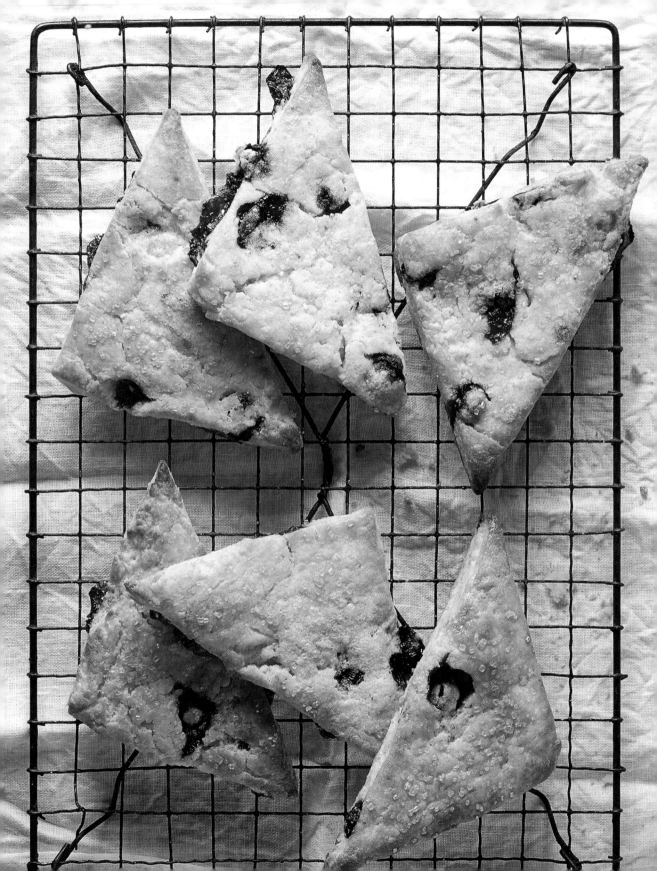

# BERRY SCONES

*Makes* 8 scones

AS WITH ANY PASTRY, THE TRICK HERE IS TO KEEP THE DICED BUTTER COLD, WHICH makes for light scones, the only sort of scones to have. I like to cut these into triangles, but rounds are lovely, too. My favorite is cranberry scones. The rich red color of the cranberries against the pale golden-brown scones makes me wish they could just sit out on my counter all day long wrapped loosely in a kitchen towel. But once you and your family experience the moist flakiness of these lightly sweet scones, you'll know why they never seem to brighten your kitchen counter for very long.

2 cups (280 g) all-purpose gluten-free flour (see page 21)

1 teaspoon xanthan gum (omit if your blend already contains it)

1 tablespoon baking powder

½ teaspoon (3 g) kosher salt

2 tablespoons (24 g) granulated sugar, plus more for sprinkling

5 tablespoons (70 g) unsalted butter, chopped and chilled

6 ounces whole berries (I love cranberries or blueberries here)

1 cup (8 fluid ounces) whole milk, chilled, plus more for brushing

PREHEAT THE OVEN TO 400°F. LINE BAKING SHEETS WITH UNBLEACHED PARCHMENT PAPER and set them aside.

In a large bowl, place the flour, xanthan gum, baking powder, salt, and sugar. Whisk to combine well.

To the large bowl with the dry ingredients, add the chopped butter and toss to coat in the dry ingredients. With a floured thumb and forefinger or the side of a large spoon, flatten each piece of butter. Add the berries to the bowl, and toss to coat. If using fresh cranberries, slice them in half before adding to the bowl.

Add the milk to the dry ingredient–butter mixture and stir to combine until the dough just comes together. Handling it as little as possible to keep the butter from melting in your hands, turn the dough out onto a lightly floured surface and pat it into a rectangle about ½ inch thick.

Cut the dough into 8 triangles. Transfer the triangles to the baking sheets lined with parchment paper, a couple of inches apart. Brush with a bit of milk and sprinkle with a tiny bit of sugar, if you like.

Bake for 15 to 20 minutes, until the scones are puffed up and slightly brown around the edges. Serve immediately.

# BLUEBERRY MUFFINS

## *Makes* 12 muffins

THESE BLUEBERRY MUFFINS ARE LIGHT, TENDER, MOIST, AND BURSTING WITH BLUEBER-ries. The buttermilk helps make them super tender, as does controlling the amount of xanthan gum. You can make them with a more traditional all-purpose gluten-free flour blend, and the end result will simply be less tender. If using frozen blueberries, to minimize the amount of blue color that bleeds into the batter, don't defrost the berries but rinse them with very cold water until the water runs clear right before adding them to the batter.

1 ¾ cups (245 g) Basic Gum-Free Gluten-Free Flour (see page 21)

½ teaspoon xanthan gum

¼ cup (36 g) cornstarch

1 teaspoon baking powder

¼ teaspoon baking soda

½ teaspoon (3 g) kosher salt

8 tablespoons (112 g) unsalted butter, at room temperature

¾ cup (150 g) granulated sugar

2 eggs (100 g, weighed out of shell), at room temperature, beaten

1 teaspoon pure vanilla extract

1 cup (150 g) fresh or frozen blueberries

1 cup (8 fluid ounces) buttermilk, at room temperature

PREHEAT THE OVEN TO 350°F. GREASE OR LINE THE WELLS OF A STANDARD 12-CUP MUFFIN TIN and set the tin aside.

In a medium-size bowl, place the flour blend, xanthan gum, cornstarch, baking powder, baking soda, and salt, and whisk to combine well. In a separate, large bowl, place the butter and granu-lated sugar, and using a handheld mixer, beat until light and fluffy. Add the eggs and vanilla, and beat until well combined.

Toss the blueberries in about 1 teaspoon of the dry ingredients, and set aside. To the butter mix-ture, add the remaining dry ingredients in 4 batches and the buttermilk in 3 batches, alternating be-tween the two and beginning and ending with the dry ingredients, mixing until just combined after each addition. The batter should be thick but soft. Fold the blueberries and reserved dry ingredients into the batter until they're evenly distributed throughout, taking care not to break the berries.

Divide the batter evenly among the prepared wells of the muffin tin. The wells will be almost completely full. Shake the pan back and forth to distribute the batter evenly in the wells. Place in the center of the preheated oven, and bake until the muffins are puffed, very, very pale golden, and firm to the touch: a toothpick inserted in the center should come out with no more than a few moist crumbs attached (about 20 minutes). Remove from the oven and allow to cool in the tin for 5 minutes before transferring to a wire rack to cool completely before serving.

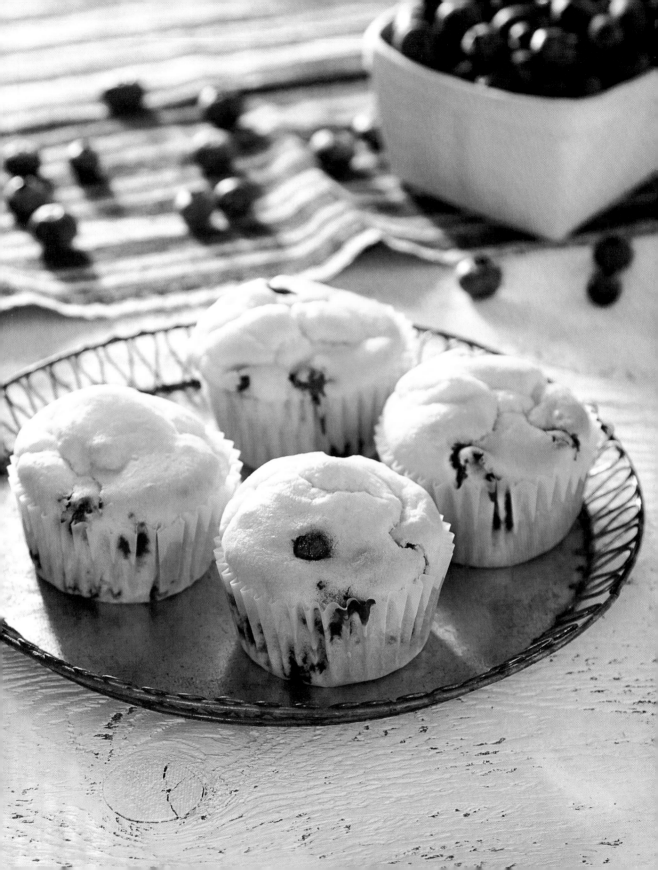

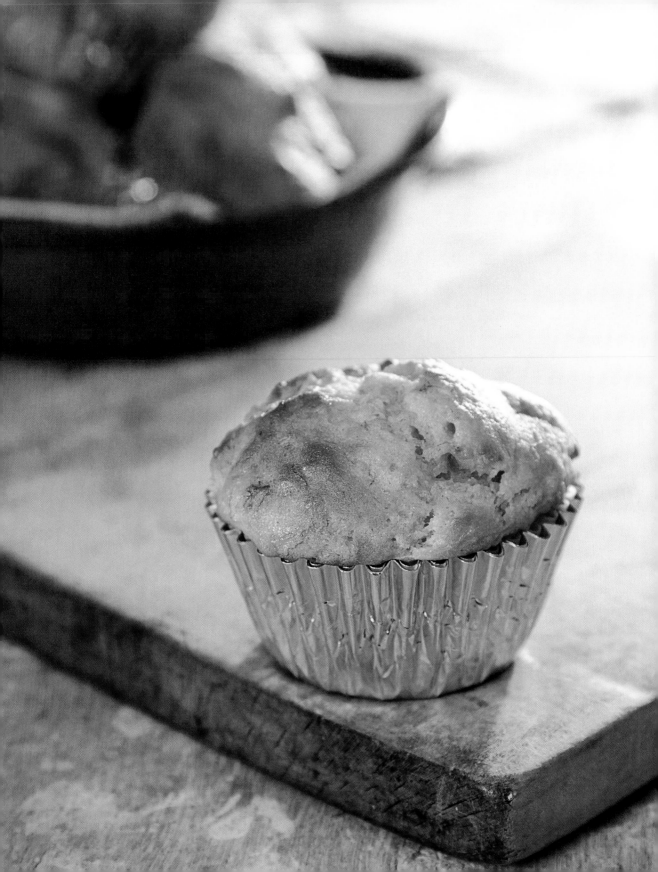

# BANANA MUFFINS

*Makes* 12 muffins

THE SECRET TO MAKING BANANA MUFFINS THAT ARE MOIST AND TENDER, AND PACKED with banana flavor, is to use less butter than usual and more bananas than you might expect. There are three mashed bananas right in the batter of these muffins. If you like some cinnamon flavor in your banana muffins, try adding 1 teaspoon of ground cinnamon to the batter. For some banana chunks, leave about ¼ of the bananas unmashed. Cut that remaining piece of banana into a small dice and fold into the batter right before baking.

1¾ cups (245 g) all-purpose gluten-free flour (see page 21)

1 teaspoon xanthan gum (omit if your blend already contains it)

1 teaspoon baking powder

½ teaspoon baking soda

⅔ cup (133 g) granulated sugar

¾ teaspoon (almost 5 g) kosher salt

6 tablespoons (84 g) unsalted butter, at room temperature

2 eggs (100 g, weighed out of shell), at room temperature, beaten

1 teaspoon pure vanilla extract

⅔ cup (5⅓ fluid ounces) buttermilk, at room temperature

1½ cups (300 g) mashed ripe bananas (from about 3 medium bananas)

PREHEAT THE OVEN TO 350°F. GREASE OR LINE THE WELLS OF A STANDARD 12-CUP MUFFIN TIN and set the tin aside.

In a medium-size bowl, place the flour blend, xanthan gum, baking powder, baking soda, sugar, and salt, and whisk to combine well. In a separate, large bowl, place the butter, eggs, vanilla, and buttermilk, and using a handheld mixer, beat until light and fluffy. To the butter mixture, add the dry ingredients, mixing until just combined after each addition. Add the mashed bananas, and mix by hand until just combined.

Divide the batter evenly among the prepared wells of the muffin tin. Shake the pan back and forth to distribute the batter evenly in the wells. Place in the center of the preheated oven and bake until the muffins are puffed and lightly golden brown and a toothpick inserted in the center comes out with no more than a few moist crumbs attached (about 20 minutes). Remove from the oven and allow to cool in the tin for 5 minutes before transferring to a wire rack to cool completely before serving.

# COFFEE CAKE

*Makes* one 9-inch cake

THIS RICH, BUTTERY SOUR CREAM CAKE IS LOVELY ON ITS OWN, BUT EVERYONE KNOWS that the real star is the crumble topping. The secret to big, generous crumbles that hold their shape during baking is to chill the raw topping until it's very firm before breaking it into irregular pieces and scattering it on the raw cake. And if you're wondering if it's OK to eat cake for breakfast, remember that it's called coffee cake because it tastes best with a big cup of coffee.

## CRUMBLE TOPPING

1 cup (140 g) all-purpose gluten-free flour (see page 21)

½ teaspoon xanthan gum (omit if your blend already contains it)

⅓ cup (73 g) packed light-brown sugar

¼ cup (50 g) granulated sugar

2 teaspoons ground cinnamon

½ teaspoon freshly grated nutmeg

½ teaspoon (3 g) kosher salt

8 tablespoons (112 g) unsalted butter, melted and cooled

## CAKE

6 tablespoons (84 g) unsalted butter, at room temperature

¾ cup (150 g) granulated sugar

2 eggs (100 g, weighed out of shell), at room temperature, beaten

1 teaspoon pure vanilla extract

1¾ cups (245 g) all-purpose gluten-free flour (see page 21)

¾ teaspoon xanthan gum (omit if your blend already contains it)

¾ teaspoon baking powder

½ teaspoon baking soda

½ teaspoon (3 g) kosher salt

1 teaspoon ground cinnamon

1 cup (256 g) sour cream, at room temperature

PREHEAT THE OVEN TO 350°F. LINE A 9-INCH SQUARE OR ROUND CAKE PAN WITH UNBLEACHED parchment paper and set it aside.

Make the crumble topping. In a medium-size bowl, place the flour, xanthan gum, brown sugar, granulated sugar, cinnamon, nutmeg, and salt, and whisk to combine, working out any lumps in the brown sugar. Add the butter, and mix to combine well. Place the bowl in the refrigerator to chill for about 10 minutes or until firm.

For the cake, in a large bowl, beat the butter and sugar until light and fluffy. Add the eggs and vanilla, blending well after each addition. Add the flour, xanthan gum, baking powder, baking soda, salt, and cinnamon, mixing well to combine after each addition. Next, add the sour cream and mix to combine. The batter will be thick.

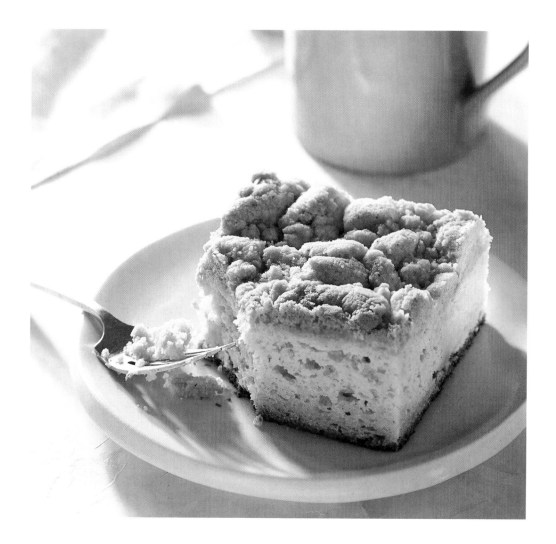

Scrape the cake batter into the prepared pan, and spread evenly with a wet spatula. Remove the topping from the refrigerator and crumble it with your fingers evenly over the batter.

Place the pan in the center of the preheated oven, and bake for approximately 35 minutes or until a toothpick inserted into the center of the cake comes out with a few moist crumbs attached. Check the cake after 25 minutes. If the topping is browning too quickly, tent the cake loosely with foil and continue baking until done. Remove from the oven and allow to cool in the pan for 10 minutes before lifting it out of the pan by the parchment paper and slicing into squares or wedges to serve.

# BREAD PUDDING

*Makes* 4 to 6 servings

BREAD PUDDING IS A CREATURE OF TOUGH ECONOMIC TIMES, WHEN NOTHING WENT to waste. And in this noble spirit of thrift, I would never use fresh gluten-free bread to make bread pudding. Not only does fresh bread make inferior bread pudding (just as it makes inferior French toast) but also fresh gluten-free bread should be enjoyed responsibly and respectfully. Bread pudding is where stale gluten-free bread is respectfully laid to rest.

¾ cup (150 g) granulated sugar

5 eggs (250 g, weighed out of shell), at room temperature, beaten

2 cups (16 fluid ounces) milk, at room temperature

2 teaspoons pure vanilla extract

3 cups cubed, stale gluten-free bread

¾ cup (164 g) packed light-brown sugar

2 tablespoons (28 g) unsalted butter, at room temperature

1 cup chopped pecans (optional)

PREHEAT THE OVEN TO 350°F. GREASE A 13 × 9-INCH BAKING DISH WITH UNSALTED BUTTER and set it aside.

In a large bowl, place the sugar, eggs, milk, and vanilla, and whisk to combine. Place the cubes of bread in the bowl, and allow to sit for a few minutes so the bread can soak up the milk mixture.

In another small bowl, combine the brown sugar, butter, and optional pecans.

Pour bread mixture evenly into the prepared baking dish. Scatter the brown sugar mixture over the top of the bread mixture. Bake for about 40 minutes, or until the eggs are set, and serve warm.

# CHEESE BLINTZES

*Makes* 9 servings

BLINTZ PANCAKES ARE THICKER AND MORE SUBSTANTIAL THAN CRÊPES (SEE PAGE 126) and can be served with either a sweet or a savory filling. There is only a touch of added sugar in the cheese filling of these blintzes, just enough to enhance the natural sweetness of the ricotta cheese. You can serve the filled pancakes without the final step of sautéing. But once you've tried the completed recipe, you'll be won over by the warmth and slight crispness that you get from sautéing and never skip it.

PANCAKES

1½ cups (12 fluid ounces) milk, at room temperature

3 tablespoons (42 g) unsalted butter, at room temperature

4 eggs (200 g, weighed out of shell) plus 1 egg white (25 g), at room temperature, beaten

1½ cups (210 g) Basic Gum-Free Gluten-Free Flour (see page 21)

½ teaspoon (3 g) kosher salt

FILLING

2 cups (250 g) low-moisture ricotta cheese, at room temperature

1 tablespoon (12 g) granulated sugar, plus more to taste

⅛ teaspoon (almost 1 g) kosher salt

4 to 5 tablespoons (56 to 70 g) unsalted butter, for sautéing

LINE A PLATE WITH UNBLEACHED PARCHMENT PAPER AND MOISTEN A TEA TOWEL UNTIL JUST damp. Set aside.

In a standard blender, place all of the pancake ingredients in the order listed. Blend until very smooth. Alternatively, you can place the milk, butter, and eggs in a large bowl and beat with a handheld mixer until smooth, and then add the flour blend and salt and beat until smooth. The batter should be the consistency of heavy cream.

Heat a heavy-bottom nonstick 9-inch skillet (or a well-seasoned and greased 9-inch cast-iron skillet) over medium heat for 2 minutes. Holding the warm skillet just above the flame, carefully ladle or pour about ¼ cup of batter right into the center of the skillet and swirl the pan to distribute the batter evenly across the entire flat surface of the pan. Cook over medium heat until the edges and underside of the pancake are lightly golden brown (about 45 seconds). With a wide spatula (and/or your fingers, carefully), flip the pancake over and cook until the other side is lightly golden brown (about another 15 seconds). Slide the pancake out of the skillet onto the parchment-lined plate. Repeat with the remaining batter. Stack the finished pancakes on top of one another, and cover with the moist tea towel to prevent them from drying out.

Place the filling ingredients in a large bowl and, using a handheld mixer, beat until whipped and smooth. Place one pancake on a flat surface in front of you, and place about ¼ cup of the filling about one-third of the way from the edge of the pancake closest to you. Fold the bottom of the pancake up over about half of the filling, fold the sides in, and roll the pancake away from you until it is closed. Repeat with the remaining pancakes and filling. If any of the blintzes are opening up, use a small dollop of filling on the edge of the pancake to seal it.

Place 1 tablespoon of unsalted butter in the heavy-bottom nonstick 9-inch skillet (or well-seasoned and greased 9-inch cast-iron skillet) and melt over medium heat. Swirl the butter around the pan, and place two filled blintzes in the pan, seam-side down. Sauté until golden brown on both sides, about 2 minutes total. Repeat with the remaining blintzes. Serve warm. The filled blintzes can also be placed on a parchment-lined baking sheet and baked in a 400°F oven for 10 minutes or until lightly golden brown.

# BISCUITS AND SAUSAGE GRAVY

*Makes* 6 servings

LIGHT AND FLUFFY BISCUITS WITH A CREAMY, RICH SAUSAGE GRAVY ARE A SOUTHERN classic. The secret to extra-flavorful gravy is to make it with the rendered fat from the cooked bulk sausage. If you clutch your pearls at the thought of cooking with sausage fat, you can drain and discard all the fat from the sausage and melt an equal amount of butter or olive oil to use in its place. And then walk that rendered sausage fat over to my house. I'll use it up.

1 recipe Buttermilk Biscuits (see page 104)

1 to 1½ pounds bulk pork sausage (or regular pork sausage with the casings removed)

¼ cup (35 g) Basic Gum-Free Gluten-Free Flour (see page 21)

¾ cup (6 fluid ounces) milk

2 tablespoons (1 fluid ounce) heavy whipping cream

1½ cups (12 fluid ounces) Chicken Stock (see page 26)

Kosher salt and freshly ground black pepper, to taste

Freshly grated nutmeg, to taste (optional)

PREHEAT THE OVEN TO 400°F. PREPARE THE BISCUIT DOUGH AND SHAPE THEM ACCORDING TO the recipe instructions. Place the shaped biscuits in the freezer to chill.

Place the sausage in a heavy-bottom skillet and cook over medium heat, breaking up any large clumps and stirring occasionally, until the sausage is lightly golden brown and cooked through. Drain the rendered pork fat away from the cooked pork and transfer it to a separate, small bowl. Remove the cooked pork from the skillet and set it aside.

Remove the baking sheet from the freezer and place it in the center of the preheated oven. Bake the biscuits until they are puffed, very fragrant, and lightly golden brown around the edges (about 20 minutes). Remove from the oven and allow the biscuits to cool briefly on the baking sheet while you make the gravy.

Return about ¼ cup of the rendered pork fat to the skillet, add the flour blend, and whisk to combine. Cook over medium heat, whisking frequently, until the mixture is light golden brown and nutty smelling (about 3 minutes, and it will go from very blond to golden brown and fragrant quite suddenly, so pay close attention). Add the milk, cream, and stock, and mix to combine. Bring the mixture to a simmer over medium heat, and cook, whisking constantly, until thickened (about 6 minutes). Stir in the salt, pepper, and the optional nutmeg to taste, add some of the cooked pork, and serve immediately over the warm biscuits.

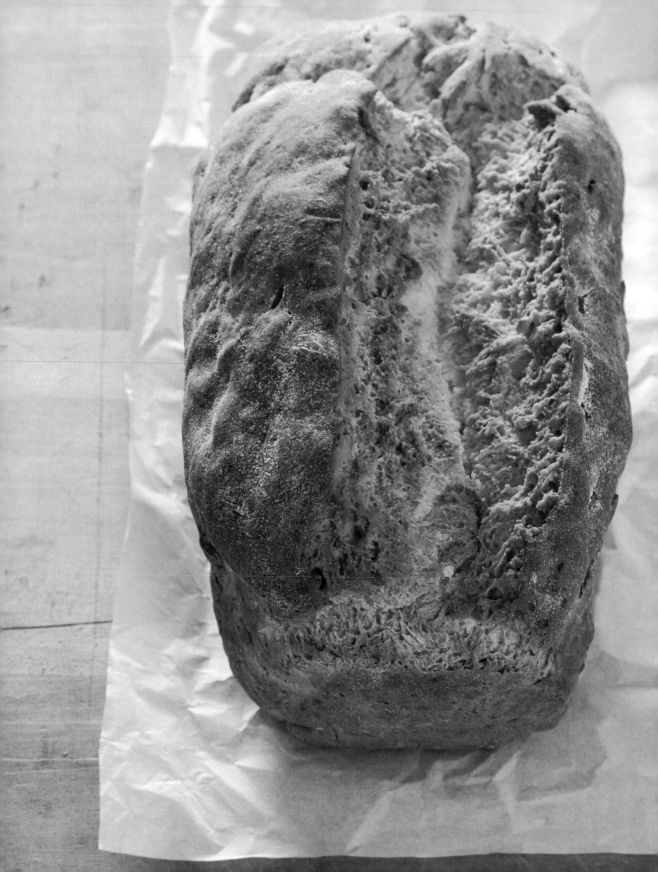

*The*

# GREATEST THING SINCE ... BREAD, GLORIOUS BREAD

SINCE THE PUBLICATION OF THE FIRST EDITION OF THIS BOOK, IN 2009, I'VE DEVELOPED A COMpletely different method and formula for baking gluten-free yeast bread. My new formula relies upon the addition of two ingredients (Expandex modified tapioca starch and whey protein isolate) to a particular all-purpose gluten-free flour. It produces yeast breads that can be handled and baked and even *taste* much like their conventional counterparts. Every shape imaginable of gluten-free bread is possible with this new style. I parlayed this new style of recipe into my third cookbook, *Gluten-Free on a Shoestring Bakes Bread*.

In this revised Shoestring edition, I have included a few of the newer style of recipes for gluten-free yeast bread. I wanted to give those readers of this book, who haven't yet baked from *Bakes Bread*, the opportunity to experience the new and exciting development in gluten-free yeast bread. However, I have kept many of the most beloved bread recipes from the first edition as is or with a few very minor modifications.

I know that many of you have relied upon these recipes for many years, and of course, nothing has changed. The recipes worked beautifully as written in 2009, and they will continue to work beautifully as written for generations to come.

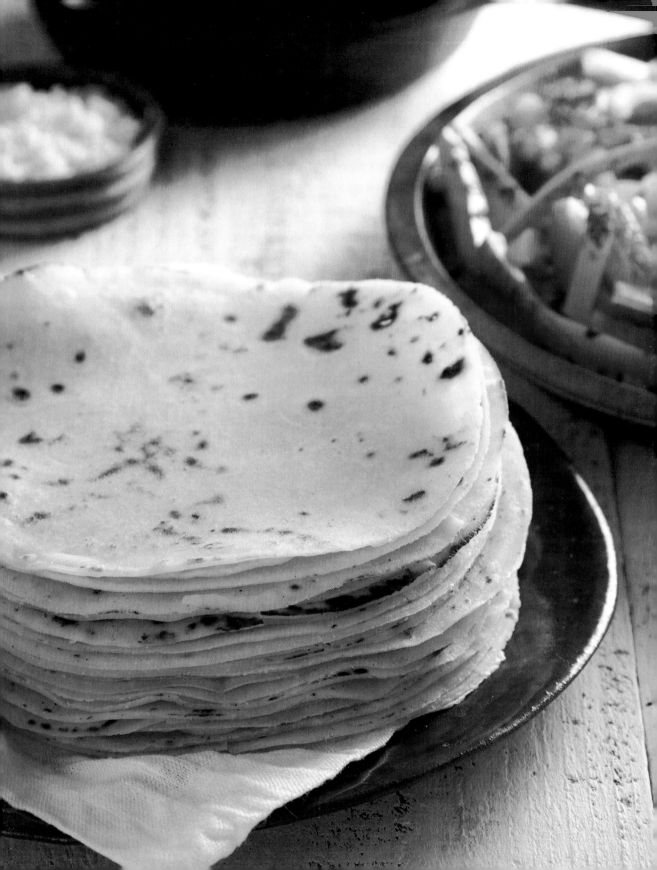

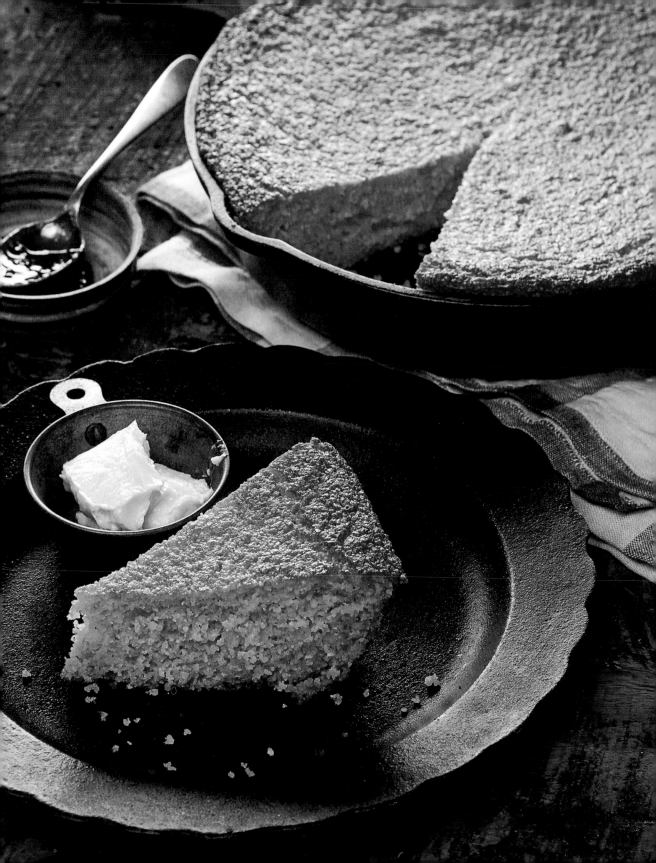

# OLD-FASHIONED CORNBREAD

*Makes* 8 servings

ORNBREAD IS A BIG FAVORITE IN MY HOUSE. CORNMEAL IS ONE OF MY HANDS-DOWN favorite gluten-free ingredients: since it's naturally gluten-free, even though I mail-order it from a source that I am sure processes it free of cross-contamination, it remains inexpensive. And because this recipe uses only cornmeal, rather than a mix of cornmeal and all-purpose gluten-free flour, the cost stays way down. So long as you keep cornmeal in your well-stocked pantry, you'll never be more than about an hour away from cornbread. It's great for Apple-Leek-Sausage Cornbread Stuffing Dinner (see page 166) or a way to complete nearly any meal. We also love it with a dollop of preserves for breakfast.

4 tablespoons (56 g) unsalted butter, melted and cooled

2 eggs (100 g, weighed out of shell), at room temperature

¼ cup (84 g) honey

1¾ cups (14 fluid ounces) buttermilk, at room temperature

2 cups (264 g) coarsely ground yellow cornmeal

1 teaspoon (6 g) kosher salt

1 teaspoon baking soda

2 teaspoons baking powder

PREHEAT THE OVEN TO 375°F. GREASE AN 8-INCH SQUARE BAKING PAN OR A 9-INCH CAST-IRON pan with unsalted butter and set it aside.

In a large bowl, place the butter, eggs, and honey, and beat until well combined. Add the buttermilk, and mix to combine well. Add the cornmeal, salt, baking soda, and baking powder, mixing well after each addition.

Pour the mixture into the prepared baking pan or cast-iron pan, place it in the center of the preheated oven, and bake for 20 to 25 minutes, until the cornbread is firm and a toothpick inserted into the center comes out clean. If you're baking in a cast-iron pan, the cornbread will likely be done in about 20 minutes.

*Shoestring* SAVINGS | ON A SHOESTRING: $4.75/cornbread
ON THE SHELF: $30/cornbread (amazing, but true)

# CORNMEAL FLATBREAD

## *Makes* 4 servings

WHEN I MAKE THIS FLATBREAD, I GENERALLY USE LIGHT COCONUT MILK, SINCE regular coconut milk has a tremendous amount of fat that I find gratuitous in this recipe. You can easily substitute another liquid for the coconut milk altogether, but it must be something with some fat or you'll have a terrible time trying to remove it from the pan. And be sure to use a pan that is at least 10 inches in diameter, or the dough will be too thick and it just won't cook all the way through. Oh, and you have to be patient and let it bake, or the center will be gooey.

2 tablespoons (28 g) extra-virgin olive oil

1 cup (140 g) all-purpose gluten-free flour (see page 21)

½ teaspoon xanthan gum (omit if your blend already contains it)

½ cup (66 g) coarsely ground yellow cornmeal

½ teaspoon (3 g) kosher salt

1 (14-ounce) can light coconut milk

PREHEAT THE OVEN TO 400°F.

Pour the olive oil in an approximately 10-inch ovenproof skillet or pan. Place the skillet or pan in a hot oven for 3 minutes, until the oil is hot. In medium bowl, whisk together the flour, xanthan gum, cornmeal, and salt. Make a well in the dry ingredients and pour in the coconut milk. Whisk to combine. The mixture should be the consistency of pancake batter.

Remove the skillet from the oven, pour the mixture into the bottom of the hot skillet, and return it to the oven.

Bake for 1 hour, until the flatbread is browned and firm to the touch. Remove from the oven, and allow the flatbread to cool briefly in the pan for a few minutes. Then slide it out, cut it into wedges, and serve right out of the oven or at room temperature.

# DINNER ROLLS

*Makes* 18 rolls

DINNER ROLLS ARE SUCH A SIMPLE PLEASURE AND ONE THAT YOU QUICKLY LEARN TO live without when you're gluten-free. Every time we go to a restaurant that isn't completely gluten-free, we're sure to ask that the waiter not bring the bread basket. We'll just have drinks. But a nice big plate of spaghetti and meatballs is taken to another level when you serve it with a beautifully browned roll on the side. Master the recipe for these dinner rolls and that simple pleasure will be yours once more, even if only in the comfort of your own home.

3 cups (420 g) Gluten-Free Bread Flour (see page 21), plus more for sprinkling

2 teaspoons (6 g) instant yeast

¼ cup (50 g) sugar

1 teaspoon (6 g) kosher salt

4 tablespoons (56 g) unsalted butter, at room temperature

1 egg (50 g, weighed out of shell), at room temperature, beaten

1 cup (8 fluid ounces) milk, at room temperature

2 tablespoons (28 g) unsalted butter, melted (for brushing)

PLACE THE FLOUR, YEAST, AND SUGAR IN THE BOWL OF YOUR STAND MIXER (OR A LARGE BOWL with a handheld mixer with dough hooks), and use a handheld whisk to combine well. Add the salt, and whisk to combine. Add the butter, egg, and milk, and mix on low speed with the dough hook(s) until combined. Raise the mixer speed to medium and knead for about 5 minutes. The dough will be quite sticky but should be smooth and stretchy. Spray a silicone spatula lightly with cooking oil spray, and scrape down the sides of the bowl. Transfer the dough to a lightly oiled bowl large enough for the dough to rise to double its size, and cover tightly with an oiled piece of plastic. Place the dough in the refrigerator for at least 1 hour and up to 3 days.

When you are ready to bake, line a small rimmed baking sheet with unbleached parchment paper and set it aside. Remove the dough from the refrigerator and turn it out onto a lightly floured surface. With the help of an oiled bench scraper, keep moving the dough as you shape it, particularly if it begins to stick to the surface or your hands. Scrape the dough off the floured surface with the bench scraper, and then fold the dough over itself. Sprinkle the dough lightly with flour, scrape the dough up again, and fold it over itself again. Repeat scraping and folding in this manner until the dough has become smoother. Keep the outside of the dough and the surface covered in a light coating of flour as you shape the dough. Handle the dough with a light touch to avoid kneading the flour into the dough, which might dry it out and result in a tight, unpleasant crumb.

With a floured bench scraper, divide the dough into 18 pieces of equal size. Working with one piece of dough at a time on a well-floured surface, flatten the dough into a disk. Pull the edges toward the center of the disk and secure the edges by pressing them between your thumb and forefinger. Turn the dough over so that the gathered edges are on the bottom, and cup your whole hands around the dough to coax it into a round shape. Place the round of dough on a lightly floured surface, and cup only one palm around the dough with the side of your hand resting on the counter (the side of your hand nearest your pinkie). Maintaining contact between the side of your hand and the surface, begin to move your hand in a circular motion while gently coaxing the edges of the dough upward (toward the top of the round) with the tips of your fingers.

Place the first roll on the prepared baking sheet. Repeat with the remaining pieces of dough, placing the rolls less than 1 inch apart from one another, in rows of 3 or 4. Cover the baking pan with oiled plastic wrap and set it aside in a warm, draft-free location to rise for about 45 minutes, or until nearly doubled in size.

About 20 minutes before the rolls have completed their final rise, preheat the oven to 350°F. Uncover the rolls and brush the tops generously with the melted butter. Place the baking sheet on the lower rack of the preheated oven, and bake until lightly golden brown and the inside of the rolls register about 185°F on an instant-read thermometer (about 20 minutes). Allow to cool briefly in the pan before serving.

If you'd like to freeze these rolls, prepare as directed, and then bake them at 300°F until they reach 170° on an instant-read thermometer (about 17 minutes). Do not brown. Allow them to cool completely before wrapping tightly and freezing. Defrost on the counter until no longer frozen solid, and then place on a baking sheet, brush with butter as directed, and finish baking at 350°F.

*Shoestring* SAVINGS | ON A SHOESTRING: 38¢/roll | ON THE SHELF: $1.00/roll

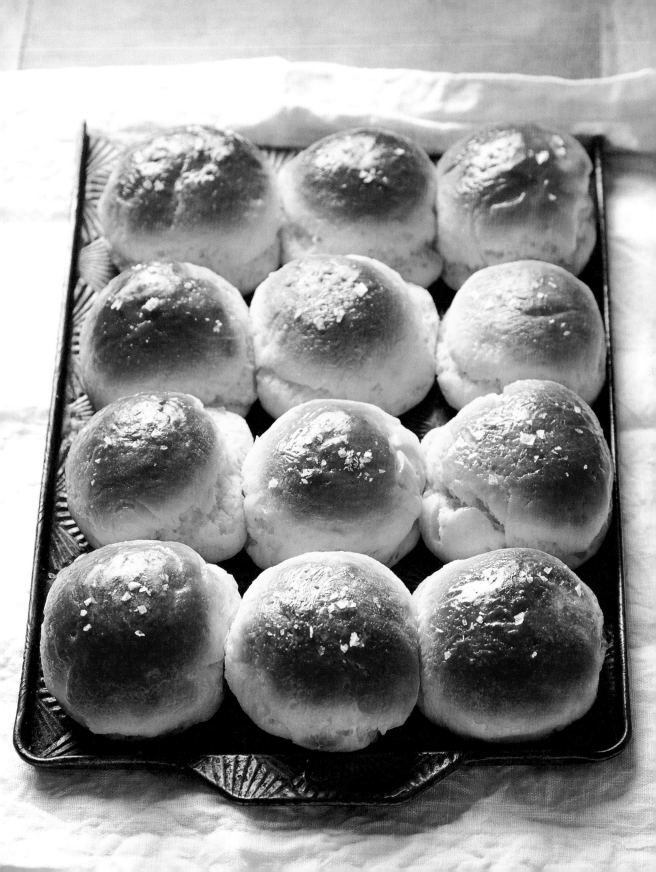

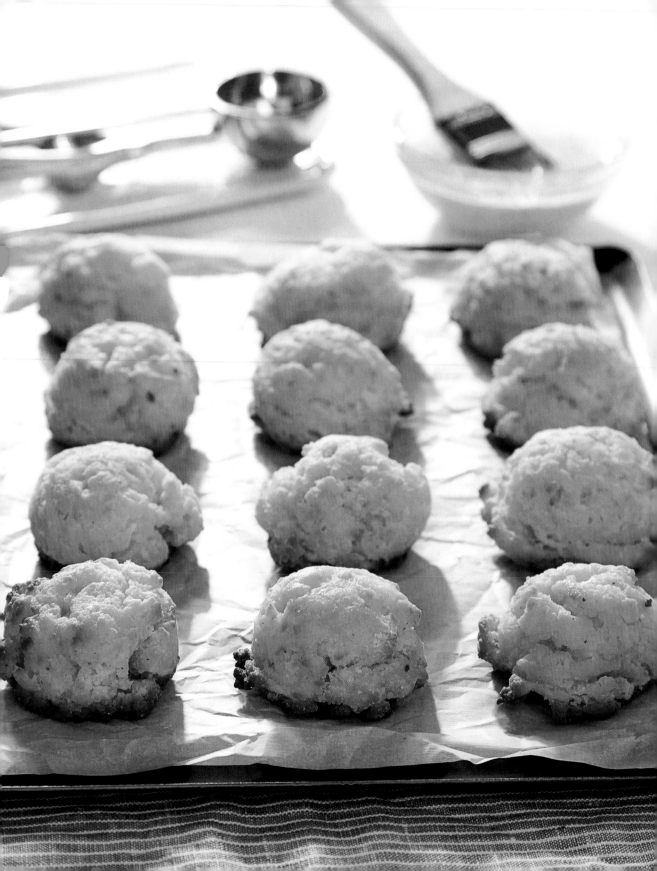

# DROP BISCUITS

*Makes* 12 biscuits

DROP BISCUITS ARE THE MOST UNFUSSY OF BISCUITS. THE DOUGH IS WETTER THAN buttermilk biscuit dough (see page 104) and is simply scooped directly from the mixing bowl onto a prepared baking sheet and baked immediately. They don't have the flaky layers of a laminated biscuit, but they're still light and fluffy and are a wonderful way to complete a meal. I often double this recipe, scoop the dough into baking sheets, and freeze in a single layer. Once frozen, I pile the shaped raw biscuits into a zip-top bag and store in the freezer. When I need a quick biscuit, I simply return them to a baking sheet and bake from frozen. Another 5 minutes or so of baking time is all it takes when baking them from frozen.

1 ¾ cups (245 g) all-purpose gluten-free flour (see page 21)

¾ teaspoon xanthan gum (omit if your blend already contains it)

¼ cup (36 g) cornstarch

1 tablespoon baking powder

¼ teaspoon baking soda

½ teaspoon (3 g) kosher salt

2 teaspoons (8 g) granulated sugar

8 tablespoons (112 g) unsalted butter, grated and chilled

1 cup (8 fluid ounces) buttermilk, chilled

1 tablespoon (14 g) unsalted butter, melted

PREHEAT THE OVEN TO 425°F. LINE A LARGE RIMMED BAKING SHEET WITH UNBLEACHED parchment paper and set it aside.

In a large bowl, place the flour, xanthan gum, cornstarch, baking powder, baking soda, salt, and sugar, and whisk to combine well. Add the grated and chilled butter, and mix to combine. Create a well in the center of the dry ingredients, add the buttermilk, and mix until just combined. Working quickly so the dough doesn't get warm, drop the batter by the ¼ cup, using two large spoons or a 2-inch ice-cream scoop, about 1½ inches apart on the prepared baking sheet. Do not pack the dough into the ice-cream scoop. Press the mounds of dough down gently to flatten the tops, and brush lightly with the melted butter.

Place the baking sheet in the center of the preheated oven and bake until lightly golden brown all over (about 15 minutes). Remove from the oven and allow to set briefly before serving.

# BUTTERMILK BISCUITS

*Makes* 8 biscuits

THESE BEAUTIES ARE LIGHT AND FLAKY AND COMFORTING ANY TIME OF DAY, LIKE A proper biscuit should be. Even better, they can be frozen after the dough is cut into rounds and then baked from frozen in a preheated 425°F oven for about 20 minutes. It's best to freeze them first on a baking sheet, so they don't clump together, and then transfer them to a freezer-safe, resealable plastic bag. These biscuits are perfect for serving with Sausage Gravy (see page 91).

1 ¾ cups (245 g) all-purpose gluten-free flour (see page 21), plus more for sprinkling

¾ teaspoon xanthan gum (omit if your blend already contains it)

¼ cup (36 g) cornstarch

1 tablespoon baking powder

½ teaspoon baking soda

2 tablespoons (24 g) sugar

1 teaspoon (6 g) kosher salt

8 tablespoons (112 g) unsalted butter, roughly chopped and chilled

1 cup (8 fluid ounces) buttermilk, chilled

PREHEAT THE OVEN TO 375°F. LINE A RIMMED BAKING SHEET WITH UNBLEACHED PARCHMENT paper and set it aside.

In a large bowl, place the flour, xanthan gum, cornstarch, baking powder, baking soda, sugar, and salt, and whisk to combine. Add the cold, chopped butter to the large bowl with the dry ingredients, and toss to coat. Place each piece of butter between your floured thumb and forefinger to flatten. Create a well in the center of the flour mixture, and pour in the buttermilk. Mix with a large spoon or spatula until the dough begins to come together.

Turn the dough out onto a lightly floured surface, dust with a bit more flour, and roll out into a thick rectangle. Fold the rectangle in half lengthwise, dust again lightly with flour, and roll the dough out again into a thick rectangle. Once more, fold in half lengthwise, and fold again widthwise to create a smaller, thicker rectangle. Dust lightly with flour, and roll out the dough into a rectangle about 1 inch thick. With a floured, round 2 ½-inch biscuit or cookie cutter, cut out rounds of dough and place them about 2 inches apart from one another on the prepared baking sheet. Gather and reroll the scraps of dough, and cut out as many more rounds as possible, placing them on the baking sheet.

Place the baking sheet in the freezer for at least 5 minutes (or in the refrigerator for at least 10 minutes) to chill the dough.

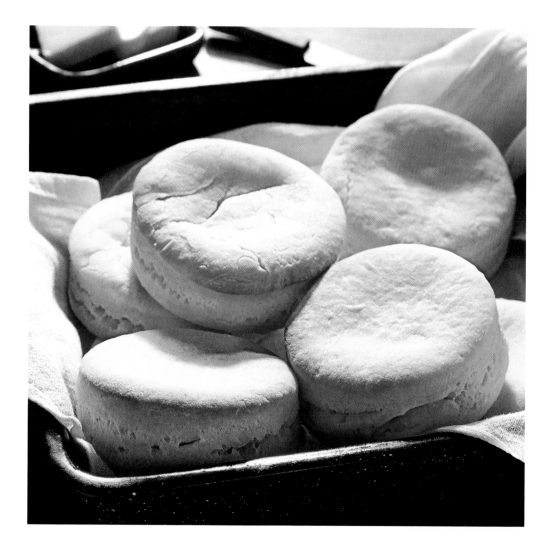

Place the chilled dough on the baking sheet in the center of the preheated oven, and bake until the biscuits are puffed and pale golden (about 15 minutes). Allow the biscuits to set briefly on the baking sheet. Serve warm or at room temperature.

I do not recommend baking and then freezing these biscuits. They are much better frozen raw and then served as freshly baked.

*Shoestring* SAVINGS | ON A SHOESTRING: 43¢/biscuit
ON THE SHELF: $2.00/biscuit

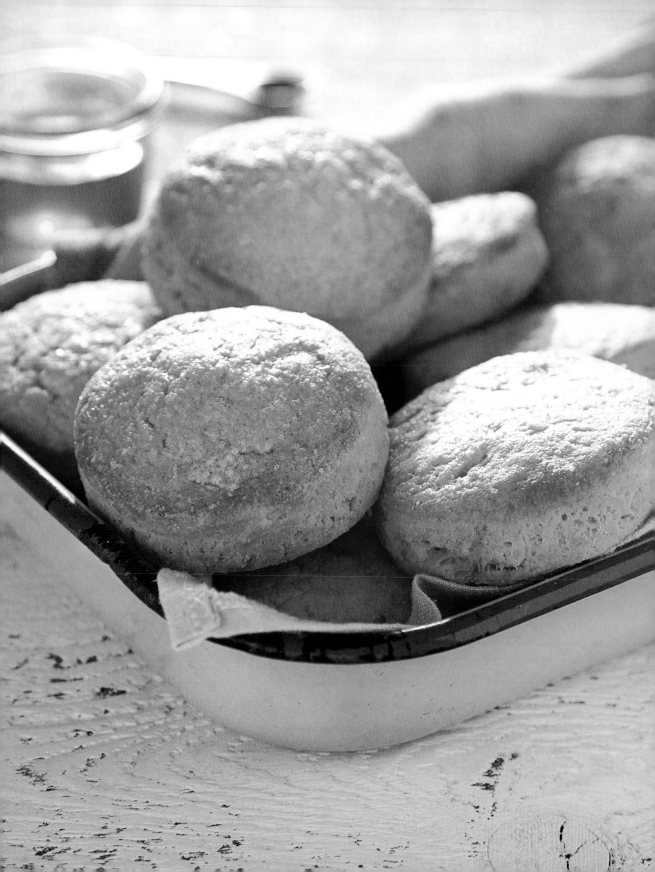

# SWEET POTATO BISCUITS

*Makes* 6 to 8 biscuits

THESE BISCUITS ARE A NEWER TWIST ON AN OLD FAVORITE. THEIR BEAUTIFUL GOLDEN color and sweet aroma never disappoint. Like the Buttermilk Biscuits (page 104), these can be placed 1 inch apart on a rimmed baking sheet and frozen before baking, and then stored in a freezer-safe bag until you're ready to use them. Just increase the baking time by about 5 minutes if you bake them from frozen, or defrost them overnight in the refrigerator before using them.

1 ¾ cups (245 g) all-purpose gluten-free flour (see page 21), plus more for sprinkling

¾ teaspoon xanthan gum (omit if your blend already contains it)

¼ cup (36 g) cornstarch

1 tablespoon baking powder

½ teaspoon baking soda

2 tablespoons (24 g) granulated sugar

1 teaspoon (6 g) kosher salt

8 tablespoons (112 g) unsalted butter, roughly chopped and chilled

¾ cup puréed baked sweet potatoes (from about 2 medium sweet potatoes, baked and peeled)

⅓ cup (85 g) sour cream, chilled

¼ cup (2 fluid ounces) milk, chilled

PREHEAT THE OVEN TO 400°F. LINE A RIMMED BAKING SHEET WITH UNBLEACHED PARCHMENT paper and set it aside.

In a large bowl, place the flour, xanthan gum, cornstarch, baking powder, baking soda, sugar, and salt, and whisk to combine. Add the cold, chopped butter to the large bowl with the dry ingredients, and toss to coat. Place each piece of butter between your floured thumb and forefinger to flatten. In a separate small bowl, place the sweet potatoes, sour cream, and milk, and mix to combine well.

Create a well in the center of the flour mixture, and pour in the sweet potato mixture. Mix with a large spoon or spatula until the dough begins to come together.

Turn the dough out onto a lightly floured surface, dust with a bit more flour, and roll out into a thick rectangle. Fold the rectangle in half lengthwise, dust again lightly with flour, and roll the dough out again into a thick rectangle. Once more, fold in half lengthwise and fold again widthwise to create a smaller, thicker rectangle. Dust lightly with flour, and roll out the dough into a rectangle about 1 inch thick. With a floured, round 2 ½-inch biscuit or cookie cutter, cut out rounds of dough and place them about 2 inches apart from one another on the prepared baking sheet. Gather and reroll the scraps of dough, and cut out as many more rounds as possible, placing them on the baking sheet.

Place the baking sheet in the freezer for at least 5 minutes (or in the refrigerator for at least 10 minutes) to chill the dough.

Place the chilled dough on the baking sheet in the center of the preheated oven and bake until the biscuits are puffed and pale golden (about 15 minutes). Allow the biscuits to set briefly on the baking sheet. Serve warm or at room temperature.

# WHITE SANDWICH BREAD

*Makes* 1 loaf

WHEN I NAILED THE RECIPE FOR THIS BREAD, I KNEW LUNCH WOULD NEVER BE the same again. As you can see in the photograph, this sandwich bread has a thick, bakery-style crust that makes a satisfying crunch when you bite into it. It's sturdy enough to stand up to any filling at all, and it doesn't need to be toasted to do it. Once it has cooled completely, it can also be sliced as thin as Melba toast, cut into rectangles, and served with cheese. Picture the sandwich you've been missing and know that the wait is over. This recipe is nearly identical to the version published in the first edition of this book. In fact, the only alteration is the substitution of instant yeast for active dry yeast. The recipe still calls for an all-purpose gluten-free flour, not my newer bread flour formula. Simply put, it wasn't broken, so I didn't feel the need to fix it.

3 cups (420 g) all-purpose gluten-free flour (see page 21)

2 ¼ teaspoons xanthan gum (omit if your blend already contains it)

2 teaspoons (12 g) kosher salt

2 ½ teaspoons (almost 8 g) instant yeast

¼ teaspoon cream of tartar

2 tablespoons (25 g) granulated sugar

1 ½ cups (12 fluid ounces) warm milk (about 95°F)

4 tablespoons (56 g) butter, melted and cooled

1 teaspoon apple cider vinegar

2 egg whites (50 g), at room temperature

GREASE OR LINE A 9 × 5-INCH LOAF PAN (OR EVEN SLIGHTLY SMALLER) AND SET IT ASIDE.

In the bowl of a stand mixer fitted with the paddle attachment, place the flour, xanthan gum, salt, yeast, cream of tartar, and sugar. Whisk together with a separate, handheld whisk.

Add the milk, butter, vinegar, and egg whites, mixing on low speed after each addition. Scrape down the sides of the mixer bowl as necessary during mixing.

Turn the mixer to medium-high speed and mix for about 3 minutes. The dough will be thick, smooth, and quite wet.

Scrape the dough into the prepared loaf pan. The dough should leave only about an inch to spare at the top of the loaf pan. Cover the dough with lightly oiled plastic wrap and allow it to rise in a warm, humid, draft-free place for 30 to 45 minutes. It should be overflowing the top of the loaf pan by at least ½ inch when you retrieve it but will not have doubled in volume. It may take longer to rise properly in colder, drier weather and less time in warmer, more humid weather.

When the dough has nearly reached the end of its rise, preheat the oven to 375°F.

Remove the plastic wrap and place the pan in the center of the preheated oven. Bake for 45 minutes to 1 hour, or until the internal temperature of the bread reaches about 195°F on an instant-read thermometer. The outside will form a thick, brown crust. Allow to cool for about 10 minutes in the pan before transferring to a wire rack to cool completely.

To freeze this bread, cool completely and then slice, wrap tightly, and freeze. Defrost as many slices at a time as you need in the toaster.

*Shoestring* SAVINGS | ON A SHOESTRING: $4.74/large loaf
ON THE SHELF: $8.00/large loaf

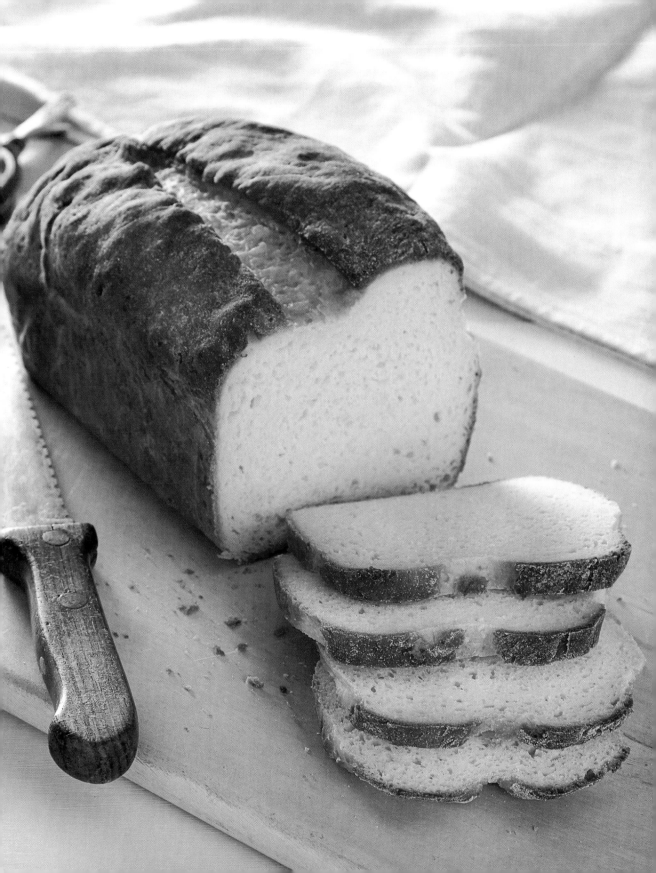

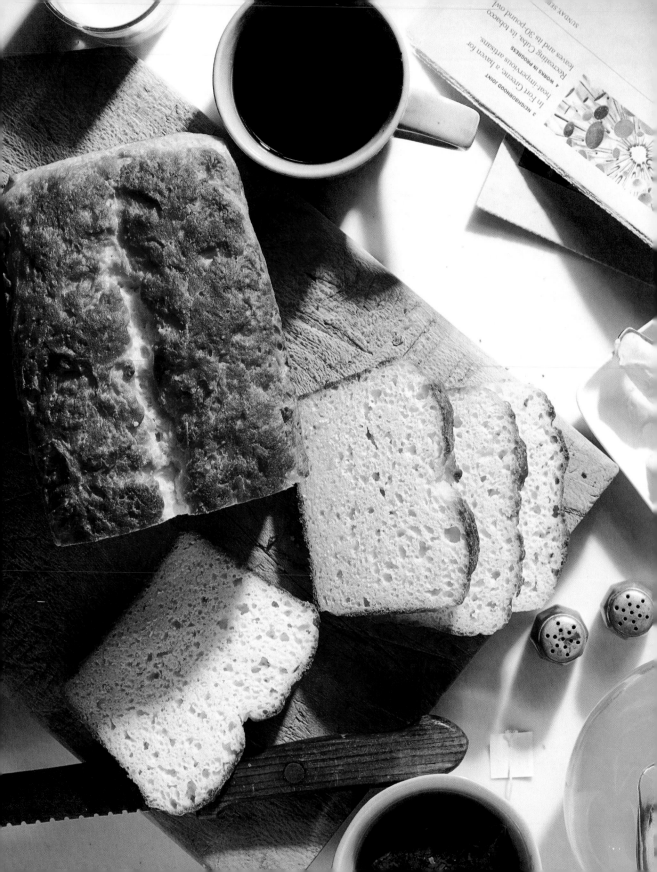

SUNDAY SE

3 NEIGHBORHOOD JOINT  4 WORKS IN PROGRESS
In Fort Greene, a haven for    Recreating Cuba, its tobacco
heat-impervious artisans.    leaves and its 30-pound owl

# ENGLISH MUFFIN BREAD

*Makes* 1 loaf

I F A WHOLE LOAF SEEMS LIKE TOO MUCH OF A COMMITMENT, THIS DOUGH CAN ALSO BE divided before baking and placed into molds to make individual English muffins. Simply reduce the baking time to 30 to 40 minutes. Sprinkling it with cornmeal, whether it's made as a loaf or as muffins, is the finishing touch that lends this recipe its authentic feel.

3½ cups (490 g) all-purpose gluten-free flour (see page 21)

2½ teaspoons xanthan gum (omit if your blend already contains it)

¼ teaspoon cream of tartar

1 tablespoon (12 g) granulated sugar

2½ teaspoons (almost 8 g) instant yeast

2 teaspoons (12 g) kosher salt

¼ teaspoon baking soda

1 teaspoon apple cider vinegar

1 egg white (25 g), at room temperature

2 tablespoons (28 g) neutral oil

2 cups (16 fluid ounces) warm milk (about 95°F)

GREASE OR LINE A 9 × 5-INCH LOAF PAN, AND SET IT ASIDE.

In the bowl of your stand mixer fitted with the paddle attachment, place the flour, xanthan gum, cream of tartar, sugar, yeast, salt, and baking soda. With a separate, handheld whisk, whisk to combine well. Add the vinegar, egg white, and oil, and mix on low speed to combine. With the mixer on low speed, add the milk in a slow and steady stream. Once the dry ingredients have mostly incorporated into the wet ingredients, turn the mixer up to medium high and mix for about 3 minutes.

Scrape the dough into the prepared loaf pan, smooth the top, and cover with a lightly oiled piece of plastic wrap. Place it in a warm, moist place to rise for 30 to 45 minutes, until the dough has risen past the lip of the loaf pan. In cool, dry weather, the dough may take longer to rise; in warm, moist weather, it may take less time to rise.

When the dough is nearing the end of its rise, preheat the oven to 375°F.

After the dough has risen, uncover the dough, and place the loaf pan in the center of the oven. Bake for 45 to 55 minutes, or until pale golden and crusty on top. The internal temperature of the bread should reach about 185°F on an instant-read thermometer. Allow the bread to cool in the pan for 10 minutes before transferring to a wire rack to cool completely.

Since this is a very moist bread, if you would like to freeze it, you'll need to slice it and then insert a small sheet of unbleached parchment paper between each slice before wrapping and freezing. Otherwise, you won't be able to separate an individual slice to defrost in the toaster.

# BRIOCHE BREAD

*Makes* 1 large loaf

THIS BRIOCHE BREAD IS A REAL TREAT. IT'S LIGHTLY SWEET AND RICH WITH EGGS AND butter. It also has a superthick golden crust and golden yellow softness inside. You'll find it makes the best French toast you've ever had, gluten-free or not, and even makes delicious sandwiches. All the eggs in this recipe make for a really puffy, stable loaf and also give this bread a long life in the refrigerator. The dough can also be used to make brioche rolls.

2 ½ cups (350 g) all-purpose gluten-free flour (see page 21)

1 ¾ teaspoons xanthan gum (omit if your blend already contains it)

½ cup (100 g) granulated sugar

1 ½ teaspoons (almost 5 g) instant yeast

1 teaspoon cream of tartar

¾ teaspoon (almost 5 g) kosher salt

1 teaspoon grated lemon zest

½ teaspoon apple cider vinegar

5 eggs (250 g, weighed out of shell), at room temperature

½ cup (4 fluid ounces) warm milk, about 95°F

10 tablespoons (140 g) unsalted butter, at room temperature

IN THE BOWL OF YOUR STAND MIXER FITTED WITH THE PADDLE ATTACHMENT, PLACE THE flour, xanthan gum, sugar, yeast, cream of tartar, and salt. With a separate, handheld whisk, whisk to combine well.

To the bowl of dry ingredients, add the lemon zest, vinegar, and eggs one at a time, and mix on low speed to combine after each addition. With the mixer on low speed, add the milk in a slow and steady stream. Once the dry ingredients have mostly incorporated into the wet ingredients, with the mixer still on low speed, add the butter 1 tablespoon at a time. Once all the butter has been added, turn the mixer up to medium-high speed and beat for about 3 minutes.

When the dough has finished mixing, scrape it into the prepared loaf pan. Cover with an oiled piece of plastic wrap, and place the pan in a warm, moist place to rise for 30 to 45 minutes until the dough has risen past the lip of the loaf pan. In cool, dry weather, the dough may take longer to rise; in warm, moist weather, it may take less time to rise.

When the dough has nearly reached the end of its rise, preheat the oven to 375°F.

After the dough has risen, remove the plastic wrap and place the loaf pan in the center of the preheated oven. Bake for 20 minutes. Then cut a slash down the center of the bread to allow steam to escape, and tent the loaf with foil. Bake 20 to 25 minutes more, or until golden brown with a thick crust on top. Allow the bread to cool in the loaf pan for about 10 minutes before transferring to a wire rack to cool completely.

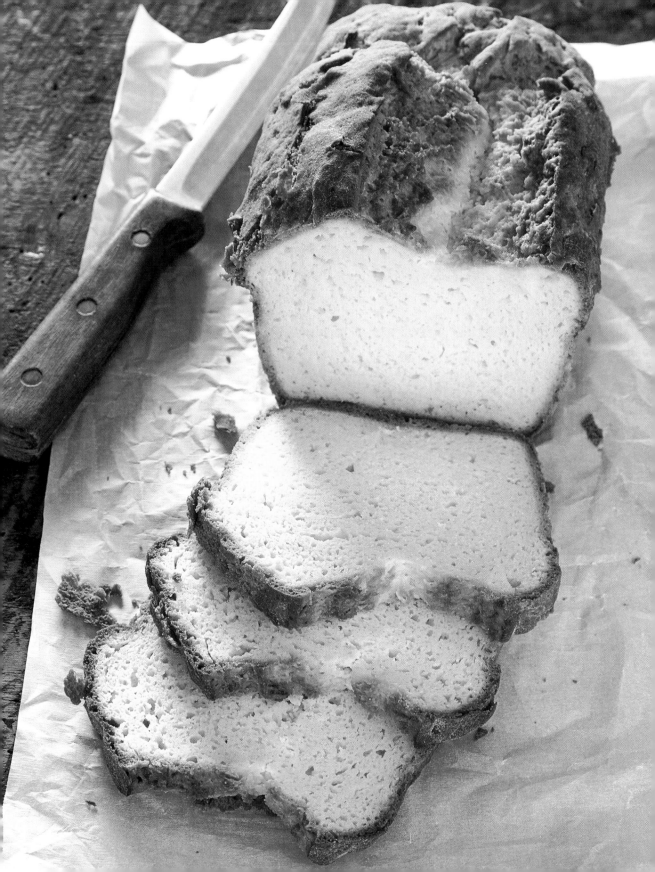

# IRISH SODA BREAD

*Makes* 1 large loaf

W E HAVE NO FAMILY CONNECTION AT ALL TO IRELAND, BUT I ALWAYS TELL my children that they can celebrate any holiday they like. They always want to celebrate St. Patrick's Day by eating Irish soda bread. I'm beginning to think that they're just in it for the food, though, and I'm not entirely sure that alone qualifies as celebrating. Irish soda bread is a little different than most other quick breads. It's made with baking soda and baking powder, like other quick breads, but it's traditionally not baked in a loaf pan, and the dough is firmer than you might expect.

4 cups (560 g) all-purpose gluten-free flour (see page 21), plus more for sprinkling

2 teaspoons xanthan gum (omit if your blend already contains it)

2¼ teaspoons baking powder

1 teaspoon baking soda

½ teaspoon (3 g) kosher salt

¼ teaspoon cream of tartar

¾ cup (150 g) granulated sugar

6 tablespoons (84 g) unsalted butter, roughly chopped and chilled

1½ to 2 cups (225 to 300 g) raisins (I like Thompson seedless raisins)

2 eggs (100 g, weighed out of shell)

1½ to 1¾ cups (12 to 14 fluid ounces) buttermilk, chilled

PREHEAT THE OVEN TO 375°F. GREASE A 9-INCH ROUND BAKING PAN AND SET IT ASIDE.

In a large bowl, place the flour, xanthan gum, baking powder, baking soda, salt, cream of tartar, and granulated sugar, and whisk to combine well. Add the chopped and chilled butter, and toss to coat the butter in the dry ingredients. Between your well-floured thumb and forefinger, flatten each chunk of butter and return it to the dry ingredients. Add the raisins (more or less, to taste), and toss to coat the raisins in the dry ingredients. In a separate bowl, add the eggs to 1½ cups of the chilled buttermilk, and beat to combine well. Create a well in the center of the dry ingredients, add the buttermilk and egg mixture, and mix gently to combine. The dough should come together. With clean hands, gather the dough gently. If there are any spots that are dry and crumbly, add more buttermilk by the tablespoon as necessary to bring the dough together.

Turn the dough out onto a lightly floured surface and sprinkle lightly with more flour. Pat the dough into a round that is approximately 9 inches in diameter, piling it higher toward the center and sprinkling lightly with more flour as necessary to prevent sticking. Place the dough in the prepared baking pan and, with a very sharp knife, slice a large X on the top about 1 inch deep (each slash should be about 6 inches long). If the dough seems to have warmed during handling, place the pan in the freezer to chill for 10 minutes or until the butter is once again firm.

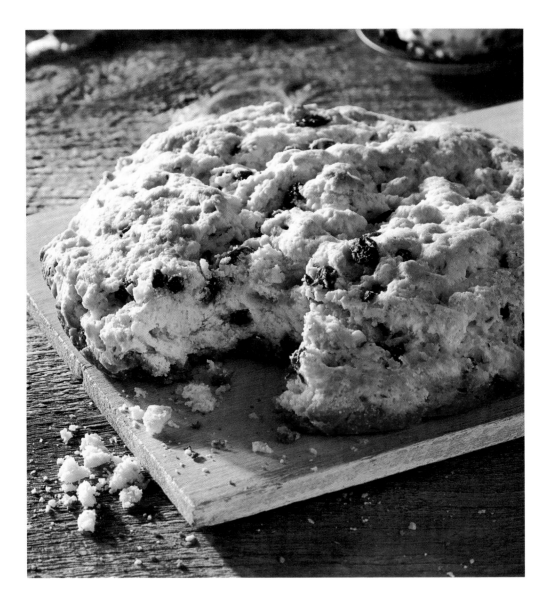

Place the baking pan in the center of the preheated oven and bake until a toothpick inserted in the center comes out clean and the bread is firm to the touch (about 45 minutes). Remove from the oven and allow to cool in the baking pan for 10 minutes before turning out onto a wire rack to cool further. Slice and serve warm, with butter. It is also excellent wrapped tightly and stored at room temperature and then served toasted the next day. Further storage is not recommended.

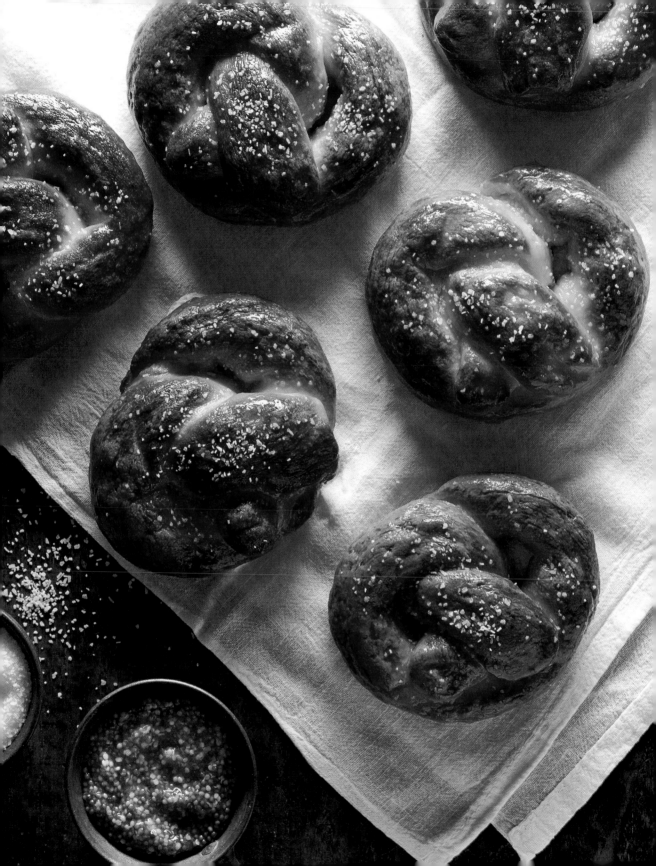

# SOFT PRETZELS

*Makes* 10 soft pretzels

THIS PRETZEL DOUGH IS VERY VERSATILE. IT CAN BE SHAPED INTO PRETZEL BITES, dinner rolls, or even hamburger buns. Whatever the shape you decide upon, though, be sure to boil the dough in a baking soda bath before baking. That keeps it from expanding too much in the oven, which keeps the pretzels nice and chewy and ensures a nice dark brown crust on the baked pretzels. My Philadelphia-born husband won't admit it, but these taste just like the soft pretzels they sell all over Philly. Yum.

3 ¼ cups (455 g) all-purpose gluten-free flour (see page 21), plus more for sprinkling

1 ½ teaspoons xanthan gum (omit if your blend already contains it)

½ cup (43 g) cultured buttermilk blend powder (or nonfat dry milk)

1 tablespoon (18 g) instant yeast

¼ teaspoon cream of tartar

¼ teaspoon baking soda

1 tablespoon (13 g) packed light-brown sugar

1 teaspoon (6 g) kosher salt

1 teaspoon apple cider vinegar

2 tablespoons (28 g) unsalted butter, at room temperature

2 egg whites (50 g), at room temperature

1 ½ cups (12 fluid ounces) warm water (about 95°F)

Baking soda bath for boiling (6 cups water plus 1 tablespoon baking soda plus 1 teaspoon salt)

Egg wash (1 egg plus 1 tablespoon water, beaten)

Coarse salt, for sprinkling

PLACE THE FLOUR, XANTHAN GUM, BUTTERMILK POWDER, YEAST, CREAM OF TARTAR, BAKING soda, and sugar in the bowl of your stand mixer fitted with the paddle attachment. With a separate, handheld whisk, whisk to combine well. Add the salt, and whisk again to combine well. Add the vinegar, butter, and egg whites, and mix to combine well. With the mixer on low speed, add the warm water in a slow but steady stream. Once you have added all the water, turn the mixer up to high, and mix for about 3 minutes. The dough will be wet. With the mixer on low speed, add more flour by the tablespoonful, 1 tablespoon at a time, until the dough starts to pull away from the sides of the bowl in spots. It should still be relatively wet but not so wet that parts of it don't clump together.

Line a large baking sheet with unbleached parchment paper. Spray the paper with nonstick cooking spray and set it aside. Turn the dough out onto a lightly floured surface. Dust the top with flour and, using a sharp knife or bench scraper, divide into 10 pieces of equal size. With wet hands, roll each piece of dough into a cylinder that is about 12 inches long and about ¾ inch thick. Twist the dough into a pretzel shape, and place it on the prepared baking sheets. Repeat with the remaining pieces of dough. Cover with oiled plastic wrap and place in a warm, draft-free environment and allow to rise until nearly doubled in volume (about 1 hour).

While the dough is nearing the end of its rise, preheat the oven to 375°F and place the baking soda bath in a large heavy-bottom pot on the stovetop to boil over high heat.

Once the dough is done rising, place the pretzels a few at a time into the boiling baking soda bath for less than a minute per side. Remove the rolls with a strainer and return them to the baking sheet. Brush each pretzel with the egg wash, and sprinkle lightly with coarse salt. Place the pretzels in the center of the preheated oven and bake until golden brown all over, about 15 minutes. Allow to cool briefly on the pan before serving.

*Shoestring* SAVINGS | ON A SHOESTRING: 48¢/pretzel
ON THE SHELF: $1.83/pretzel (frozen)

# FLOUR TORTILLAS

*Makes* 10 to 15 tortillas,
depending upon size

FOR FAR TOO LONG, I USED COMMERCIALLY PREPARED CORN TORTILLAS WHENEVER I made burritos, quesadillas, and anything in between. I figured gluten-free flour tortillas were going to be way more trouble than they were worth. Boy, was I wrong. They have precious few ingredients, and I even make them in a dry cast-iron skillet, so there's little clean-up. It's nice to have an authentic burrito now and then. It makes a great lunchbox item for my kids, too.

If you don't have Expandex modified tapioca starch, you can replace it in this recipe with an equal amount, by weight, of regular tapioca starch/flour.

1 ¾ cups (245 g) all-purpose gluten-free flour (see page 21), plus more for sprinkling

35 grams (about ¼ cup) Expandex modified tapioca starch

½ teaspoon baking powder

1 teaspoon (6 g) kosher salt

4½ tablespoons (54 g) vegetable shortening

¾ cup (6 ounces) warm water (about 85°F)

IN A LARGE BOWL, PLACE THE FLOUR, EXPANDEX, BAKING POWDER, AND SALT, AND WHISK TO combine. Add the vegetable shortening and toss it in the dry ingredients. With the tines of a large fork, break up the shortening into small pieces about the size of small peas. Create a well in the center of the mixture, and add most of the water. Mix to combine. The dough will come together and be thick. If there are any crumbly bits, add the remaining water by the teaspoonful. Knead the dough together and press it into a ball, cover with a moist tea towel, and allow to sit for about 20 minutes. The dough will stiffen a bit as it absorbs more of the water.

Heat a 10- or 12-inch cast-iron skillet over medium-high heat. Divide the dough into five pieces. Begin with one piece of dough, and cover the rest with a moist tea towel to prevent them from drying out. On a lightly floured surface, with a rolling pin, roll out the first piece of dough until it is ⅛ inch thick. Cut out as many rounds as you can (should be three or four) with a 6- or 8-inch metal cake cutter. The lid of a pot that is about the same size will also work. Stack the raw tortillas on top of one another, dusting lightly with flour between them, if necessary, to prevent them from sticking. Gather the scraps and set them aside. Repeat with the remaining pieces of dough, including gathering and rerolling all of the scraps together.

Once all the tortillas have been rolled out and cut, place them one at a time in the center of the hot skillet and cook on one side until bubbles begin to appear on the top surface and the tortilla darkens in color a bit on the underside (about 45 seconds). Flip the tortilla over with a wide spatula, and cook on the other side until more bubbles form and the tortilla darkens on the underside (about another 45 seconds). Remove the tortilla from the pan, place on a moist tea towel, and cover gently. Repeat with the remaining tortillas.

If you don't plan to use the tortillas right away, place them, still wrapped in the towel, in a plastic bag to seal in the moisture. Use within a few hours.

*Shoestring*
SAVINGS | ON A SHOESTRING: 26¢/each
ON THE SHELF: 87¢/each

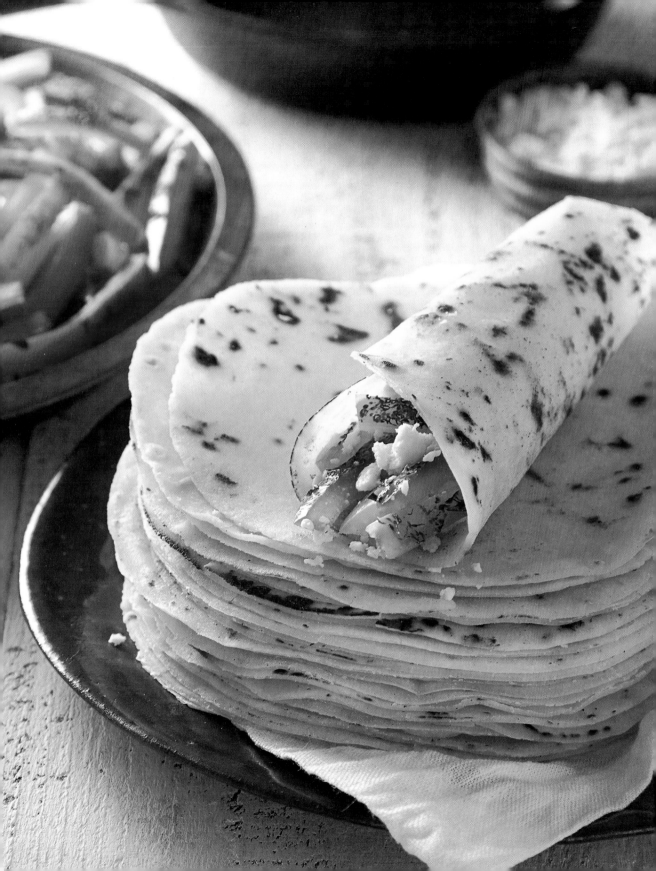

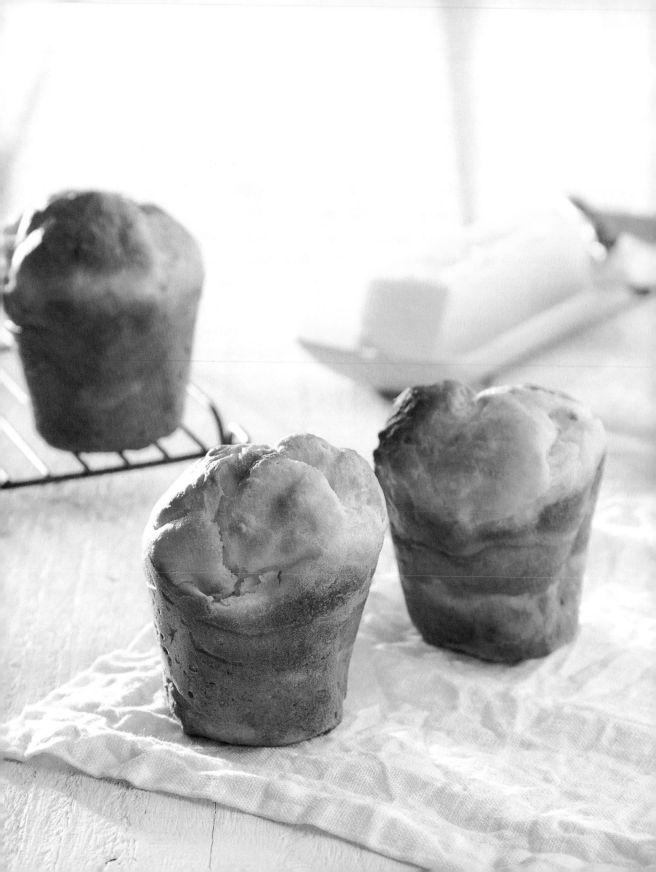

# POPOVERS

*Makes* 6 large or 12 small popovers

IF YOU'VE NEVER HAD POPOVERS, YOU'VE BEEN MISSING OUT. CRUSTY ON TOP, ALMOST pudding-like at the very bottom, they're super easy to make, require very few ingredients, and you can even use a plain old muffin tin. Although using a special popover pan does make a more beautiful presentation, and the spacing between the cups helps them to puff, you can live your whole life without a popover pan very nicely, thank you. If you would like to use one of my recommended all-purpose gluten-free flour blends, like Better Batter, you will need 1⅔ cups (13⅓ fluid ounces) milk. Omit the xanthan gum if the blend you use already contains it.

1½ cups (210 g) Basic Gum-Free Gluten-Free Flour (see page 21)

¼ teaspoon xanthan gum

¾ teaspoon (almost 5 g) kosher salt

2 tablespoons (28 g) unsalted butter, melted and cooled

3 eggs (150 g, weighed out of shell), at room temperature, beaten

1¼ cups (10 fluid ounces) milk, at room temperature

PREHEAT THE OVEN TO 400°F. GREASE WELL A 6-CUP POPOVER PAN (OR A REGULAR MUFFIN tin with very deep wells) with unsalted butter and set it aside.

In a large bowl, whisk together the flour, xanthan gum, and salt. Add the butter, eggs, and milk, whisking well after each addition until the batter is smooth.

Place the greased popover pan in the hot oven for 2 minutes. Remove from the oven, and immediately fill the wells of the pan ¾ of the way full. Return the pan to the oven and bake for 20 minutes. Turn the oven down to 325°F, and continue baking until lightly golden brown on top (about another 10 minutes). Serve immediately, plain, with butter, or with your favorite jam or preserves.

# CRÊPES

*Makes* 20 crêpes

RÊPES ARE SIMILAR TO BLINTZ PANCAKES (SEE PAGE 89) BUT MORE DELICATE AND savory, as they're thinner and have lovely, lacy edges. The batter can easily be made ahead of time and even makes the best crêpes when it's been resting in the refrigerator for a bit prior to cooking. You don't need a special crêpe pan or roller. You just need a nonstick skillet and a spatula.

1 ¾ cups (245 g) Basic Gum-Free Gluten-Free Flour (see page 21)

½ teaspoon (3 g) kosher salt

3 eggs (150 g, weighed out of shell), at room temperature, beaten

2 tablespoons (28 g) unsalted butter, melted and cooled

2 cups (16 fluid ounces) milk, at room temperature

IN A LARGE BOWL, PLACE THE FLOUR AND SALT, AND WHISK TO COMBINE WELL. IN A SEPARATE, small bowl, place the eggs, butter, and milk, and whisk to combine well. Create a well in the center of the flour and pour in the wet ingredients. Whisk until very well combined. The batter will thicken a bit as you whisk.

For the very best results, cover the bowl and place the batter in the refrigerator overnight or for up to 2 days. Before using the batter, remove it from the refrigerator, whisk until smooth, and allow it come to room temperature. You can use the batter immediately, though. It should be about the consistency of half-and-half (thicker than milk, thinner than heavy cream). Transfer the batter to a large spouted measuring cup.

Line a plate with unbleached parchment paper and set aside.

Heat a heavy-bottom nonstick 9-inch skillet (or a well-seasoned and lightly greased 9-inch cast-iron skillet) over medium heat for 2 minutes. Holding the warm skillet just above the flame, carefully pour about 5 tablespoons (a bit more than ¼ cup) of batter right into the center of the skillet, and swirl the pan to distribute the batter evenly across the entire flat surface of the pan. Once you get a rhythm going, you should be able to begin swirling as soon as the first drop of batter hits the pan. Cook over medium heat until the edges and underside of the crêpe are lightly golden brown (about 60 seconds). With a wide spatula (and/or your fingers, carefully), turn the crêpe over and cook until the other side is lightly golden brown (about another 45 seconds). Slide the crêpe out of the skillet onto the parchment-lined plate. Repeat with the remaining batter, stacking the finished crêpes on top of one another.

The crêpes may be covered well with a moist towel and kept at room temperature for about 2 hours until you are ready to serve them, or wrapped tightly in freezer-safe wrap and frozen until ready to use. Defrost at room temperature, and refresh the crêpes in a warm, nonstick skillet for a few moments per side, per crêpe.

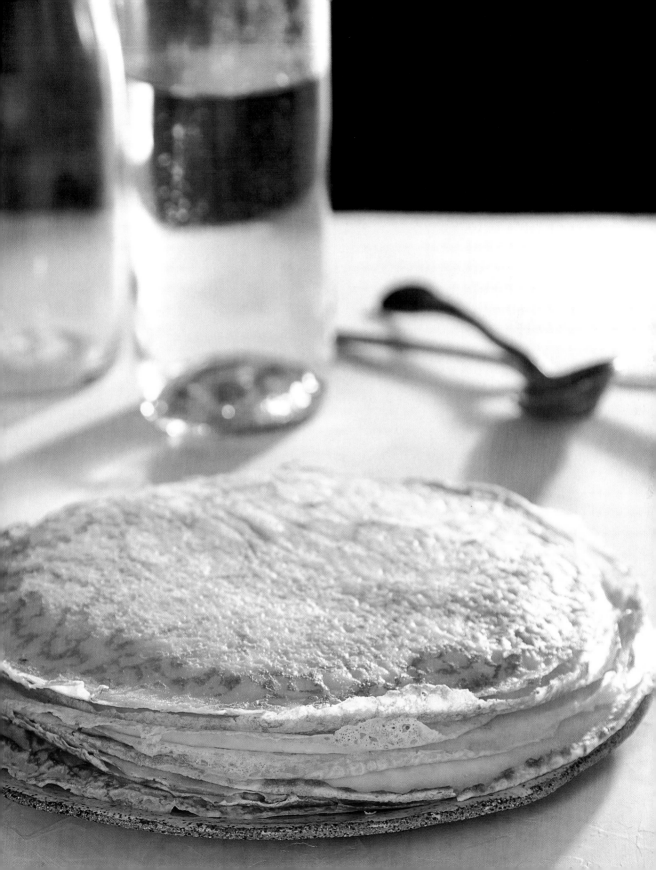

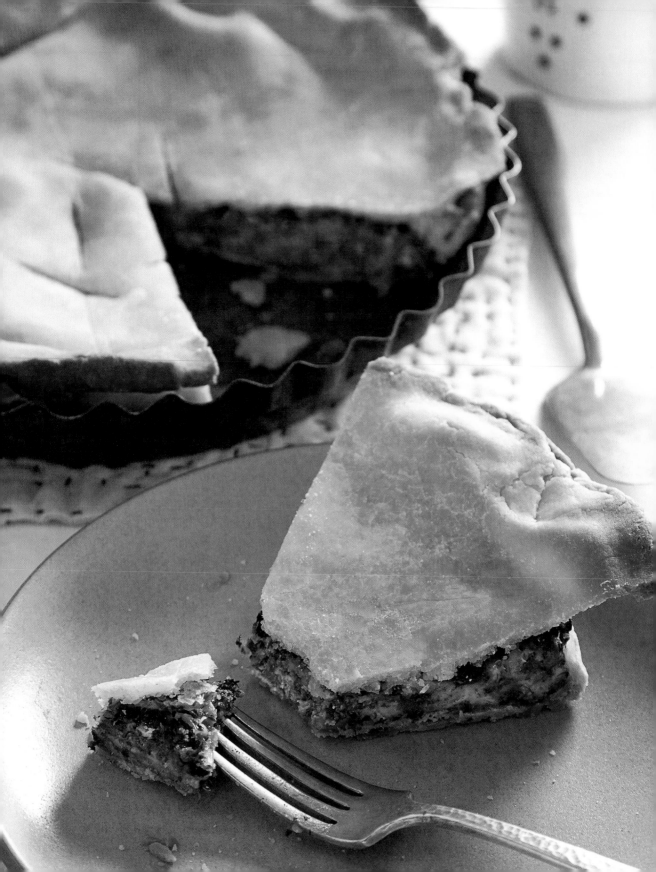

# EAT YOUR VEGETABLES: MEATLESS MEALS *and* SIDES

# CORN AND ZUCCHINI FRITTERS

*Makes* 6 servings

I DON'T KNOW ABOUT YOU, BUT WHERE I LIVE, ZUCCHINI ARE ABOUT THE EASIEST, MOST foolproof things to grow in a home garden. They're hearty and prolific, which means they nearly compensate for my lack of gardening skill. And they make such beautiful, edible flowers. I love to cook 'em with some oil, chopped onion, and chopped canned tomatoes. Zucchini really do shine when you fry them up into fritters with some flour, butter, whole kernels of corn, and a few other basic pantry items. I squeeze the shredded zucchini dry by placing it in a fine mesh bag, like a nut milk bag, or rolling it up in a tea towel and squeezing vigorously until dry.

1 egg (50 g, weighed out of shell), at room temperature, beaten

½ cup (4 fluid ounces) milk, at room temperature

2 tablespoons (28 g) unsalted butter, melted and cooled

1 cup (140 g) all-purpose gluten-free flour (see page 21)

½ teaspoon xanthan gum (omit if your blend already contains it)

1 teaspoon baking powder

½ teaspoon (3 g) kosher salt

10 ounces frozen corn kernels (or two ears of fresh corn, boiled until tender, then cut from the ear)

2 medium zucchinis, grated and squeezed dry

Vegetable oil, for frying

IN A LARGE BOWL, PLACE THE EGG, MILK, AND BUTTER, AND BEAT UNTIL WELL COMBINED. ADD the flour, xanthan gum, baking powder, and salt, and mix until well combined. Gently stir in the corn kernels, still frozen, and the grated zucchini.

Line two plates with paper towels and set aside.

In a heavy pot with at least 3-inch sides, heat about ¼ inch vegetable oil over medium-high heat until it shimmers. Drop the fritter batter by heaping tablespoons into the hot oil. Flatten each fritter with a spoon or spatula, and fry it until it turns golden brown, at least 4 minutes total, turning over the fritters once during frying.

Gently remove the fritters from the oil and drain on the lined plates. Serve immediately.

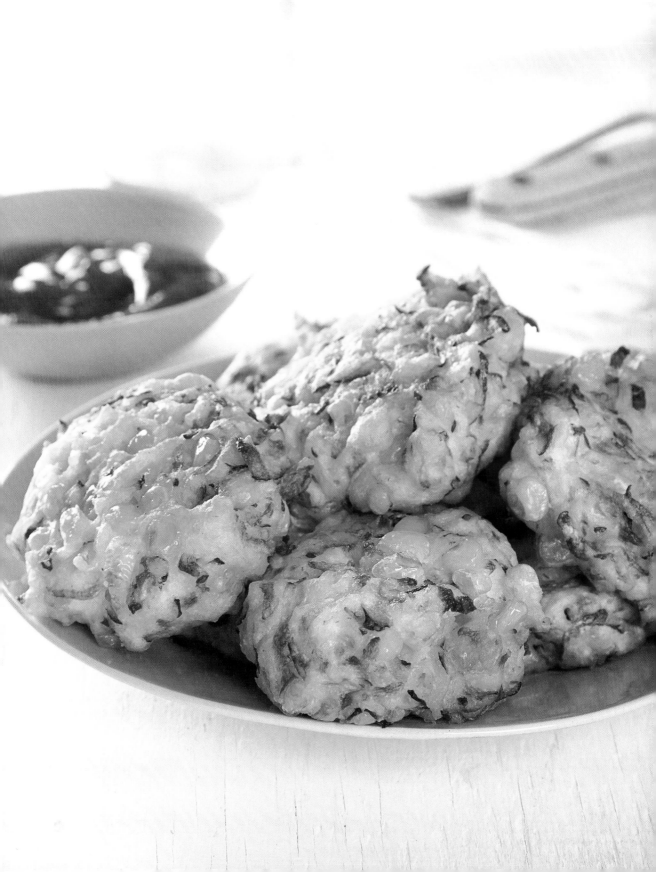

# SWEET AND SOUR BEETS

*Makes* about 4 cups sliced beets

WHY BUY PREPARED BEETS? THEY ARE SO COSTLY TO BUY ALREADY PREPARED AND terribly easy to prepare on your own. Chopped, they make a lovely addition to any salad and pair beautifully with a salty cheese, like feta. And this sweet and sour marinade is great for pickling tomatoes, cucumbers, and even hard-boiled eggs. But remember: You don't pickle pickles—they're already pickled.

3 to 4 medium-size raw beets

½ cup (4 fluid ounces) apple cider vinegar

½ cup (100 g) granulated sugar

⅛ teaspoon (almost 1 g) kosher salt

¼ teaspoon ground cinnamon

PREHEAT THE OVEN TO 375°F. DO NOT WASH THE BEETS, SINCE THAT WILL CAUSE THEM TO steam when you put them in the oven. You want them to bake dry. Trim the greens ½ inch from the top of each beet and clean them with a dry paper towel. Wrap each beet separately and tightly in aluminum foil. Place the beets in the preheated oven, and bake for 60 to 75 minutes, or until they are still firm but can be pierced easily with a fork.

Remove the beets from the oven and allow them to cool until you are able to handle them. Unwrap each beet and peel the skin off. It should come off easily. If you are particularly concerned about staining your fingers, use rubber gloves. The stain will come off readily if you wash your hands promptly after handling the beets. Slice the beets about ⅛ to ¼ inch thick and set them aside.

In a medium saucepan, place the vinegar, sugar, salt, and cinnamon, and stir to combine. Bring the mixture to a simmer over medium-high heat, stirring occasionally to ensure that the sugar dissolves in the vinegar. Gently place the sliced beets in the saucepan, return to a simmer, and cook, uncovered, for about 5 minutes.

Place the beets and all of the liquid into a sealed glass container. They will marinate and only get better over time.

# GLAZED CARROTS

*Makes* 4 to 5 side-dish servings

To make quick work of this recipe, complete the first step, blanching the carrots, 1 day ahead. These carrots are a bit sweet but balanced nicely with just enough acidity that you know it's still dinner, not dessert. Serve it at Thanksgiving or any old time. Hey, better this than candied yams.

2 pounds carrots, peeled and cut on the diagonal into ½-inch pieces

2 tablespoons (28 g) neutral oil

1 cup (8 fluid ounces) vegetable stock

½ cup (168 g) honey

2 tablespoons balsamic vinegar

½ teaspoon (3 g) kosher salt

Freshly ground black pepper, to taste

2 tablespoons (28 g) unsalted butter

BLANCH THE CARROTS BY PLACING THEM IN A MEDIUM-SIZE POT OF BOILING WATER FOR 2 minutes. Remove carrots from the boiling water and place them in a bath of ice and water for 2 minutes. Then drain them of all water with a sieve, or simply remove them from the ice bath with a slotted spoon and blot them with a towel. If you decide to make this recipe in stages, stop here and store the blanched carrots in an airtight container overnight in the refrigerator. Pick up with the next step the following day.

In a large skillet, cook the carrots in the oil over medium-high heat for 2 minutes, until they begin to brown. Add the stock, honey, vinegar, salt, pepper, and butter to the skillet, and mix to combine. Bring the mixture to a boil, and then reduce the heat and allow the mixture to simmer, stirring occasionally, until the sauce is thickened, about 5 to 6 minutes. Serve warm or at room temperature.

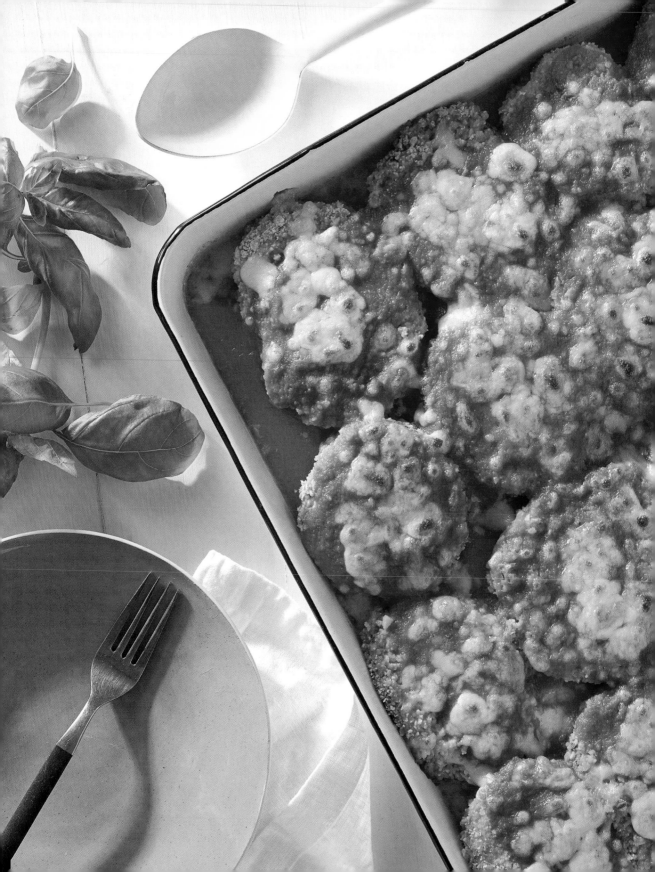

# BAKED EGGPLANT PARMESAN

*Makes* 4 main or 6 side-dish servings

THIS RECIPE MAKES A TRADITIONAL, LAYERED EGGPLANT PARMESAN. BUT IF YOU'RE feeling adventuresome or you're simply tight on time, it can be streamlined by peeling the eggplant and then cutting it into a large dice rather than slicing it. This way, rather than carefully coat each individual eggplant slice in egg and then breadcrumbs, you can simply toss the diced eggplant first in the egg mixture, sprinkle with the breadcrumbs, and bake on a rimmed baking sheet in a single layer until the eggplant is soft and the breadcrumbs are beginning to crisp. Then proceed mostly as indicated below, layering the tomato sauce, baked eggplant, and cheese and baking as directed.

Either way, it's delicious, much less messy and less time consuming than frying the eggplant before layering and baking, and considerably healthier.

2 eggs (100 g, weighed out of shell)

¼ cup (2 fluid ounces) milk

About 3 cups (360 g) panko-style gluten-free breadcrumbs

1 large or 2 medium eggplants, peeled

and sliced in ¾-inch-thick rounds

3 cups Easy Homemade Tomato Sauce (see page 48)

12 ounces low-moisture mozzarella cheese, grated

PREHEAT THE OVEN TO 400°F. LINE RIMMED BAKING SHEETS WITH UNBLEACHED PARCHMENT paper and set them aside.

Place the eggs in one wide, flat bowl, add the milk and ¼ cup (2 fluid ounces) water, and beat well. Place the breadcrumbs in another wide, flat bowl. Place one slice of raw eggplant in the egg mixture, invert it to coat the other side, and allow the excess to drip off. Next, press both sides of the eggplant firmly into the breadcrumbs and transfer to the prepared baking sheet. Repeat with the remaining slices of eggplant, arranging them 1 inch apart on the prepared baking sheets.

Place the baking sheets in the preheated oven, and bake until soft to the touch and golden brown, 15 to 20 minutes. Halfway through baking, flip the slices so they brown evenly on both sides.

While the eggplant is baking, grease a 12 × 9-inch baking dish and spoon just enough tomato sauce into the pan to cover the bottom with a thin layer. Once the eggplant is done baking, allow the eggplant to cool for 5 minutes, or even less. This allows the eggplant to become somewhat firm. Lower the oven temperature to 350°F.

Place one layer of eggplant over the layer of tomato sauce, cover each slice with sauce, and top generously with grated cheese. Continue with another layer of eggplant slices, sauce, and grated cheese, followed by one final layer.

Bake for 15 to 20 minutes, until the cheese is melted and the sauce is bubbling.

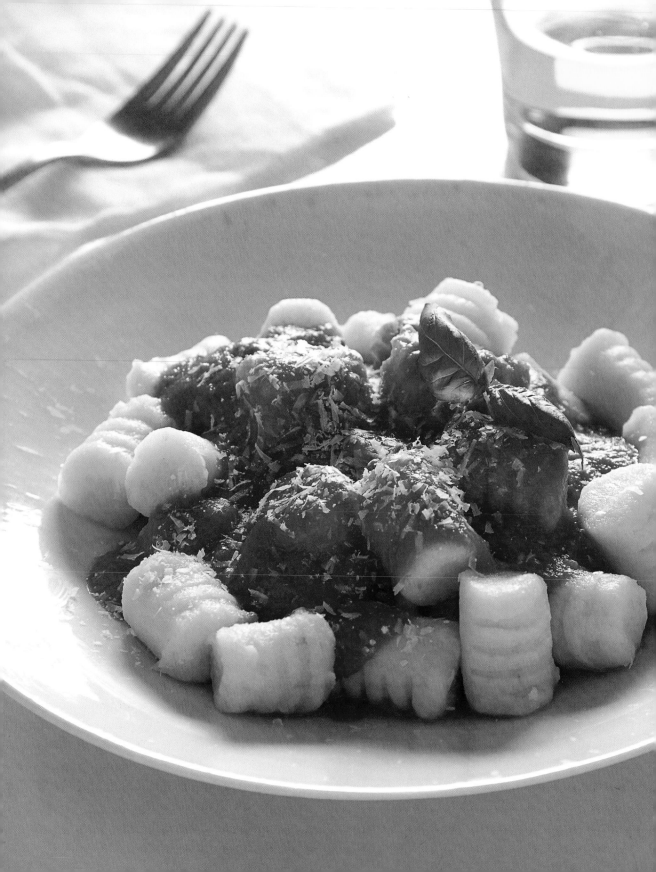

# POTATO GNOCCHI

*Makes* 4 servings

FOR THE SAKE OF SANITY (WHICH I HIGHLY PRIZE AND FIND TO BE IN SHORT SUPPLY), I suggest that you bake the potatoes for this recipe in advance. Whenever you're using the oven for something else already, bake the potatoes and keep them in the refrigerator until you are ready to use them.

Many recipes for gnocchi call for boiling the potatoes. I think that is just silly. They absorb too much moisture that way, and then you have a heck of a time combating the extra moisture in the final product. If you bake them in a dry, hot oven, you will have them just where you want them.

The recipe below assumes that you have no chilled mashed potatoes on hand. But just think of how good it would feel to be able to skip right to making the gnocchi dough. Since this recipe can be easily doubled, I often do just that and then, without boiling them, freeze half the gnocchi on a baking sheet in a single layer before putting them in a resealable freezer-safe storage bag. No need to defrost the dumplings before boiling them when you're ready to use them. Just boil them right out of the freezer.

4 large russet (or similar size) potatoes

2 tablespoons (28 g) unsalted butter, melted and cooled

1 cup (140 g) all-purpose gluten-free flour (see page 21), plus more for shaping

½ teaspoon xanthan gum (omit if your blend already contains it)

½ teaspoon (3 g) kosher salt

PREHEAT THE OVEN TO 400°F. WASH, PIERCE, AND BAKE THE POTATOES IN THEIR SKINS FOR about an hour, or until they're soft when you squeeze them. Let them cool slightly, then peel them. I use a vegetable peeler but a carefully wielded sharp knife will do. Place the skinned potatoes in a large bowl, add the butter, and then mash them until they're very smooth. If you have a potato ricer or food mill, use it to mash the potatoes until smooth. Place the mashed potatoes in the refrigerator to chill for at least 30 minutes.

Once the potatoes are chilled, add the flour, xanthan gum, and salt to the potatoes, kneading in the dry ingredients, squeezing the dough as you go. It should hold together.

Now it's time to roll the dough into ropes about 3 to 6 inches long, or as long as you can manage them. Give each lump of dough a good squeeze in between your palms, and then roll the dough either between your palms or with your palms on a floured surface, pushing away from your body. The most important thing is that the dough holds together solidly. After you have rolled a few ropes, let them sit for a few minutes. It will allow the flour mixture to absorb the moisture of the potatoes.

While the dough is sitting, boil a large pot of water. Once the water has boiled, cut the ropes into 1-inch pieces with a sharp knife, and then mark each with the tines of a fork to make ridges (which will allow the gnocchi to hold on to sauce better). One by one (and in batches of about 20), gently drop each little nugget into the boiling water, and allow the gnocchi to cook for about 3 minutes, until they float to the top (and it's very, very exciting when they do float to the top). Remove the gnocchi with a slotted spoon and set them aside. Repeat this process with the remaining dough.

Serve gnocchi with tomato sauce (or whatever else you like). The raw gnocchi can be frozen in a single layer on a baking sheet, then sealed in an airtight container. Boil them from frozen, simply adding a minute or so to the boiling time.

*Shoestring* SAVINGS | ON A SHOESTRING: 55¢/serving
ON THE SHELF: $2.07/serving

# RICOTTA GNOCCHI

*Makes* 4 servings

COMPARED TO POTATO GNOCCHI (SEE PAGE 137), RICOTTA GNOCCHI ARE SIMPLER TO make because you are spared that first step of baking, peeling, and cooling the potatoes. Just like potato gnocchi dough, ricotta gnocchi dough must hold together firmly or it will fall apart during boiling. When in doubt, stick the dough in the refrigerator, as it will become firmer as it chills. A light touch in shaping the gnocchi is the key to having delicate, and not tough, dumplings. It also keeps you from incorporating too much flour into the dough during the process. This is, unfortunately, one of those recipes where nondairy substitutes will just not work.

1¼ cups (175 g) all-purpose gluten-free flour (see page 21), plus more for shaping

½ teaspoon xanthan gum (omit if your blend already contains it)

½ teaspoon (3 g) kosher salt

3 ounces Parmigiano-Reggiano cheese, finely grated (about 1 cup)

1 egg (50 g, weighed out of shell), at room temperature, beaten

1 pound (16 ounces) low-moisture ricotta cheese

Extra-virgin olive oil, for sautéing

Easy Homemade Tomato Sauce, for serving (see page 48)

Fresh or dried herbs, for serving

IN THE BOWL OF A FOOD PROCESSOR, PLACE ALL OF THE INGREDIENTS IN THE ORDER IN WHICH they are listed. Pulse until the mixture begins to come together. Turn the food processor on high and process until the mixture is thick and well combined. Turn it out onto a lightly floured flat surface, sprinkle lightly with more flour, and pat into a disk. Cover tightly with plastic wrap, and place the dough in the refrigerator to chill for 10 minutes.

Once the dough has chilled, remove the plastic wrap and place on a lightly floured surface. Using a sharp knife or a bench scraper, cut off pieces of dough and roll them into rounds that are about 1½ inches in diameter, sprinkling lightly with more flour to prevent sticking.

Using the fingers of both hands and pushing away from your body, roll each round into a rope of dough about 6 inches long and about ¾ inch thick. Be careful not to push down on the dough, but rather roll it out. Sprinkle lightly with additional flour as necessary.

Using a sharp knife or bench scraper, cut the ropes of dough into 1-inch-long pieces. Mark the top of each piece with the floured tines of a fork to make ridges. Continue to flour the tines of the fork as necessary to prevent sticking.

To cook the gnocchi, drop them in batches in generously salted boiling water. The gnocchi will float after they have been boiling for about 2 minutes. Continue to boil for another 2 minutes before removing with a strainer. Allow most of the water to drain out of the strainer before placing the cooked gnocchi in a bowl and tossing them with a bit of olive oil to prevent the gnocchi from sticking to one another.

Instead of boiling the gnocchi, they can be sautéed in small batches in a light coating of hot olive oil in a large, heavy-bottom saucepan over medium-high heat until golden brown (about 2 minutes per side).

Serve with tomato sauce and fresh or dried herbs. The raw gnocchi can be wrapped tightly and frozen in a single layer on a baking sheet, then sealed in an airtight container. Boil them from frozen, simply adding a minute or so to the boiling time.

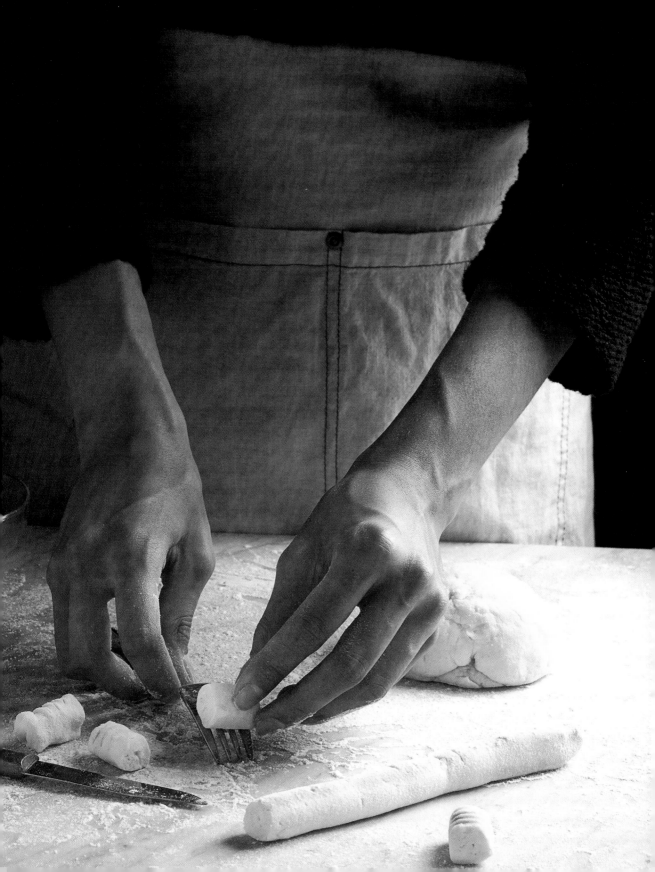

# SPINACH AND CHEESE RAVIOLI

*Makes* about 24 ravioli

THE ONLY SPECIAL EQUIPMENT YOU REALLY NEED TO MAKE RAVIOLI IS A METAL RAVIOLI cutter. It cuts and seals the ravioli all in one motion and costs only a couple dollars at any good kitchen supply store (or on the Internet). But you don't need fancy mats and rolling pins to roll out the pasta; the rest of your regular equipment will do (until you open that Italian restaurant, of course).

1 recipe Fresh Pasta Dough (page 35)

8 ounces frozen chopped spinach, thawed and squeezed dry

1 tablespoon (18 g) plus ½ teaspoon (3 g) kosher salt

8 ounces low-moisture ricotta cheese

1 ounce Parmigiano-Reggiano cheese, finely grated

2 ounces part-skim mozzarella cheese, grated

2 tablespoons chopped fresh basil

1 egg (50 g, weighed out of shell), at room temperature, beaten

⅛ teaspoon freshly ground black pepper

Egg wash (1 egg plus 1 tablespoon water, beaten)

DIVIDE THE FRESH PASTA DOUGH INTO FOUR EQUAL PORTIONS AND ROLL EACH PORTION between two sheets of plastic wrap into a rectangle ⅛ inch thick (the thickness of a nickel). Set aside the dough.

Place the spinach in a clean kitchen towel and wring out all the liquid. Begin to boil a large pot of water. Once the water is boiling, add 1 tablespoon of the salt.

While the water is coming to a boil, in a large bowl, place the ricotta cheese, Parmesan-Reggiano cheese, mozzarella cheese, basil, and spinach, and mix until well combined. Add the beaten egg, the remaining ½ teaspoon salt, and the pepper, and mix to combine. In a separate small bowl, beat the egg and water together for the egg wash and set it aside.

Slice each rectangle of pasta dough into strips that are slightly wider than the width of your ravioli cutter. Gently score each strip of pasta dough with the ravioli cutter to help you approximate where to put the filling.

Place a tablespoon of filling in the center of each scored ravioli in one strip of pasta. Brush the egg wash on all of the exposed areas along the strip of dough that are not covered by the filling. This will seal the raviolis closed. Gently place another strip of pasta squarely over the top of the first strip, pressing between ravioli. Using the ravioli cutter, cut and seal each ravioli by positioning the cutter where the dough was scored, pressing down firmly, and popping the ravioli out of the cutter with your index finger. Repeat the process with the remaining dough and filling.

Divide the ravioli into two batches. Place the first batch into the large pot of boiling water. Return the water to boiling. Cooking times will depend somewhat upon the size of the ravioli but should range from 6 to 8 minutes from the time the water begins to boil again. The ravioli are generally done once they have begun to swell in size a bit. Repeat with the second batch.

Gently remove the ravioli from the water and serve immediately with sauce. Do not rinse the ravioli or the sauce will not cling to them.

The raw ravioli can be shaped and filled and frozen in a single layer on a lined baking sheet, then sealed in an airtight container. Boil them from frozen, simply adding a minute or so to the boiling time.

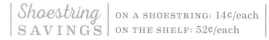

*Shoestring*
SAVINGS | ON A SHOESTRING: 14¢/each
| ON THE SHELF: 52¢/each

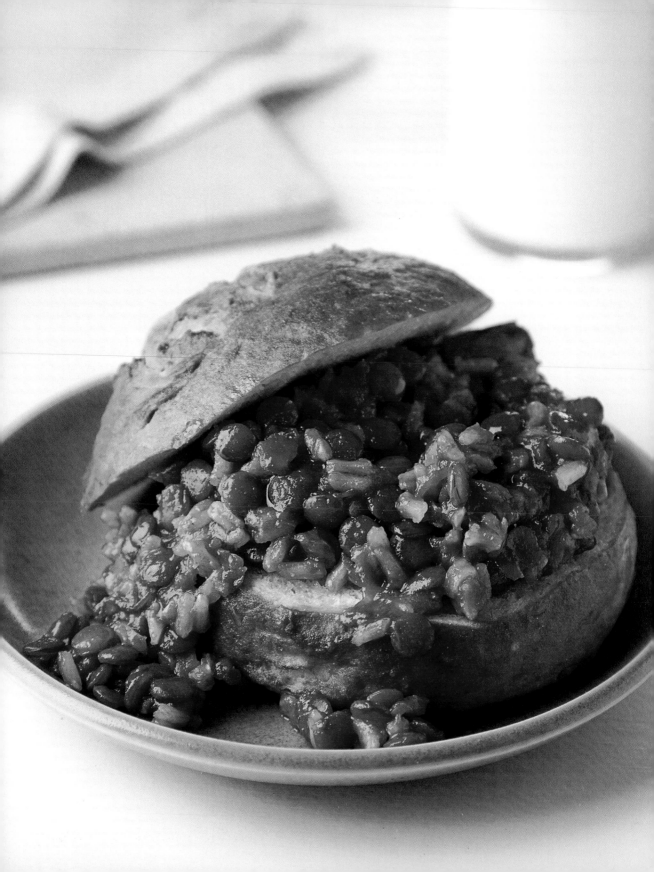

# LENTIL SLOPPY JOES

*Makes* 6 servings (as a sandwich)
or 4 servings (in a bowl)

M Y HUSBAND AND I LOVE LENTIL SLOPPY JOES, WHICH ARE NEARLY IDENTICAL TO the traditional beef version—although my children, for the most part, refuse to eat this. But I'm convinced that it's only because they made a pact in a former life that they would reject lentils for all eternity. There is no other reason that makes sense to me. To serve the sloppy Joes, you can use buns made from Dinner Rolls (page 99) simply by dividing the dough in that recipe into 8 pieces of equal size, rather than 18. The mixture is also delicious in a bowl with a dinner roll riding shotgun.

2 medium yellow onions, peeled and chopped

2 tablespoons (28 g) vegetable oil

¼ teaspoon (almost 2 g) kosher salt

⅛ teaspoon freshly ground black pepper

1½ cups dried lentils

2½ cups Easy Homemade Tomato Sauce (see page 48)

3 to 4 cups (24 to 32 fluid ounces) vegetable stock

⅔ cup (145 g) packed light-brown sugar

3 to 4 tablespoons gluten-free Worcestershire sauce

2 to 3 cups cooked brown rice

IN A LARGE STOCKPOT, SAUTÉ THE ONIONS IN THE OIL OVER MEDIUM HEAT UNTIL THEY ARE translucent, about 6 to 7 minutes. Add the salt and pepper. Add the lentils, tomato sauce, 3 cups of the vegetable stock, brown sugar, and Worcestershire sauce to the pan. Stir to dissolve the sugar and combine the rest of the ingredients. Bring the pot to a boil over medium-high heat. Reduce the heat to a simmer, cover, and cook for about 30 minutes, until the lentils are tender.

Once the lentils are tender, uncover the pot, add the rice, and stir to combine. Continue to cook, uncovered, for about another 10 to 15 minutes, until the mixture reduces and thickens. It will thicken more as it cools. If necessary, you can add more vegetable stock to achieve the right consistency.

EAT YOUR VEGETABLES: MEATLESS MEALS AND SIDES

# SPINACH PIE

*Makes* one 9-inch spinach pie

I LOVE THIS DISH FOR BRUNCH AS A GREAT ALTERNATIVE TO QUICHE. SERVE IT WITH SOME fresh fruit or some fluffy scrambled eggs. Or add some tomato sauce to the spinach mixture and it becomes more of a Mediterranean pizza, and dinner is ready to go. The olive oil crust can be made ahead of time, but it can be ready in a flash anyhow.

1 recipe Savory Olive Oil Crust (see page 33)

2 tablespoons (28 g) extra-virgin olive oil

2 garlic cloves, crushed whole and peeled

1 medium yellow onion, peeled and chopped

16 ounces frozen chopped spinach, thawed

4 ounces part-skim mozzarella cheese, grated

2 ounces Parmigiano-Reggiano cheese, grated

4 ounces feta cheese, crumbled

LINE A RIMMED BAKING SHEET WITH UNBLEACHED PARCHMENT PAPER AND SET IT ASIDE. Separate the olive oil crust into two equal portions. Place one portion between two sheets of unbleached parchment paper, and roll into a round about 10 inches in diameter. Repeat with the other portion. Place both olive oil crusts, still between sheets of parchment paper, flat on a shelf in the refrigerator to chill for 10 to 15 minutes.

While the crust is chilling, make the filling. Heat the olive oil in a small, heavy-bottom skillet over medium heat. Sauté the whole crushed cloves of garlic and onion in the oil until the onion is translucent and the garlic is fragrant, about 6 minutes. Spoon the onions and oil into a large bowl. Discard the garlic. Place the spinach in a clean kitchen towel or in a fine mesh bag, like a nut milk bag, and wring out all the liquid. Once the spinach is dry, add it to the onion and oil and mix to combine. Add the three cheeses to the spinach and onion mixture and mix well to combine thoroughly.

Preheat the oven to 350°F.

Take both crusts from the refrigerator. Remove the parchment from 1 round of dough and place it, flat, on the prepared baking sheet. Spoon the spinach mixture onto the center of the dough on the baking sheet and spread it out evenly over the surface of the dough, leaving a 1-inch border all around. From the other round of dough, remove one sheet of parchment and place it, exposed-side down, on top of the spinach mixture and squarely atop the bottom crust. Carefully remove the remaining piece of parchment from the top crust. Pinch together the edges of the top and bottom crusts all along the perimeter of the pie. With a very sharp knife, slice three to four vents into the top of the crust to allow steam to escape during baking.

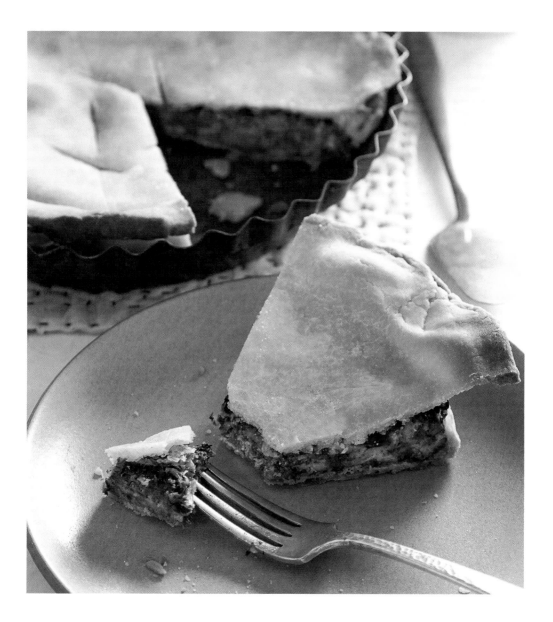

Place in the center of the oven and bake for about 30 minutes, or until nicely browned all over.

Once the pie has finished baking, remove it from the baking sheet and place on a cutting board. With a large serrated knife, slice the pie into wedges and serve immediately.

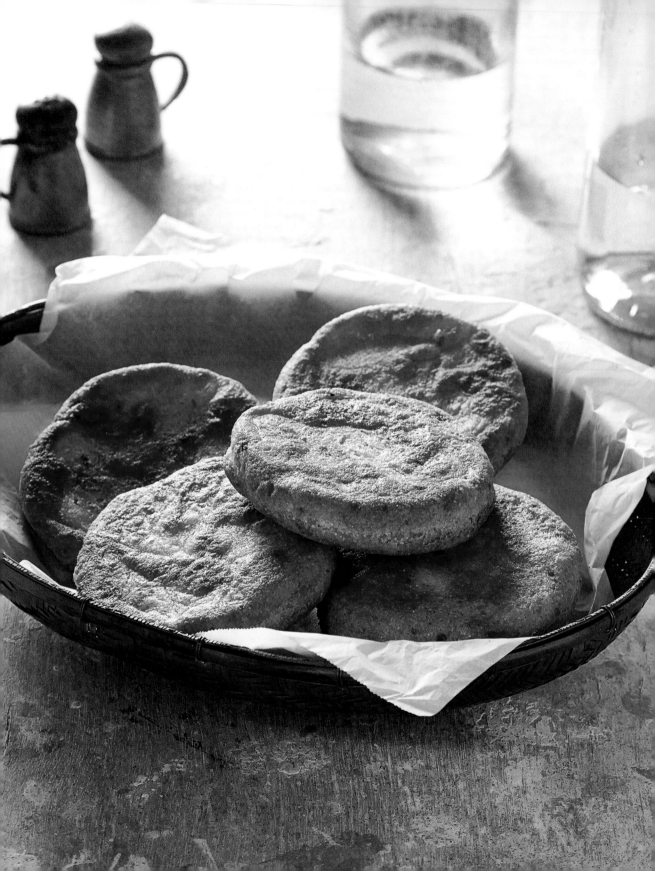

# AREPAS

## *Makes* 10 to 12 arepas

REPAS ARE BAKED OR FRIED CORNMEAL CAKES THAT ARE POPULAR IN COLOMBIA and Venezuela. They're usually served split in half and filled with something yummy, like eggs and salsa. To make them, you will need precooked cornmeal. The quintessential brand is Harina P.A.N. Making arepas is more art than science. I have tried to make the process as transparent as possible in these directions, but there is no substitute for experience. Just keep in mind that even when they do not become puffy because there's a crack you didn't seal, they still taste delicious. And practice makes perfect.

1 cup (116 g) masa harina corn flour

4 ounces part-skim mozzarella cheese, grated

⅛ teaspoon kosher salt

1 cup plus 2 to 4 tablespoons (9 to 10 fluid ounces) lukewarm water

¼ cup (56 g) vegetable or other neutral oil

IN A LARGE BOWL, PLACE THE CORN FLOUR, CHEESE, AND SALT, AND MIX TO COMBINE. ADD 1 cup of water, and stir to combine, incorporating the water into the flour mixture. Add more water by the tablespoonful if necessary for the dough to come together. Once the dough has come together, cover the bowl with plastic wrap and allow it to stand at room temperature for 3 to 4 minutes. The corn flour will continue to absorb water, and the dough will stiffen as it stands.

After the dough has stiffened, wet your hands and divide the dough into 10 to 12 portions of about 3 tablespoons each. With wet hands again, form the first piece of dough into a ball, then flatten into a disk about 2½ inches wide and ¼ inch thick by patting the dough back and forth between your open palms, like clapping. Repeat with each piece of dough.

Pour the oil into a 12-inch skillet with at least 2-inch-high sides, and heat the oil over medium-high heat until it shimmers. While the oil heats, prepare the first portion of dough for frying. Wet your hands again and press all around the edge of the disk, eliminating any cracks. Flatten along the side, smoothing as you go. When you fry the arepas, if you have successfully eliminated all cracks, steam will build up inside and they will puff and swell. It takes some practice, but it's well worth the effort.

When the oil is ready, place each portion of dough carefully in the pan and fry until golden brown, turning over once during frying and frying for 4 to 5 minutes per side. Do not crowd the pan. Fry in batches.

Drain arepas on paper-towel-lined plates before serving. With a wet serrated knife, slice the arepas in half horizontally and serve warm or at room temperature.

# CRISPY ASIAN-STYLE TOFU

*Makes* 4 servings

I OFTEN BAKE TOFU BY SIMPLY TOSSING IT WITH KOSHER SALT, FRESHLY GROUND BLACK pepper, and olive oil and then baking it in a single layer in a 400°F oven for about 15 minutes, or until the edges begin to brown. Then I pair it with fried rice and broccoli crowns, and dinner is served. When that starts to become humdrum, I go the extra mile and soak the tofu in an Asian-style marinade before baking it, as in this recipe.

½ cup gluten-free soy sauce or tamari

¼ cup plus 2 tablespoons rice vinegar

¼ cup (84 g) honey

2 tablespoons (28 g) sesame oil

2 tablespoons (28 g) vegetable or other neutral oil

1 cup (8 fluid ounces) vegetable stock

1 tablespoon fresh ginger, minced

1 (14-ounce) block extra-firm tofu

2 tablespoons (18 g) cornstarch

MAKE THE SAUCE FIRST BECAUSE YOU WILL DRY THE TOFU AND THEN SOAK IT IN THE SAUCE. In a medium saucepan, place the soy sauce, vinegar, honey, oils, vegetable stock, and ginger, and whisk well to combine. Over medium-high heat, bring the sauce to a boil. Lower the heat and, stirring constantly, allow the sauce to simmer until it has begun to reduce and thicken. Remove the sauce from the heat, transfer it to a medium-size flat bowl, and allow it to cool for at least 10 minutes.

Remove the tofu from its package, drain it, and wrap it in a clean kitchen towel. Gently but firmly squeeze the tofu in the towel to remove as much water as possible. Remove the tofu from the towel and slice it into cubes about ¾ inch square. Place the cubes into the bowl with the cooled sauce, and allow them to marinate at room temperature for at least 45 minutes to an hour. If the cubes are not covered completely by the sauce, turn them a few times while they marinate.

Preheat the oven to 350°F. Line a large, rimmed baking sheet with aluminum foil and spray it with nonstick cooking spray. Once the tofu has finished marinating, with tongs or clean fingers, carefully remove each piece of tofu from the marinade and place all of them on the prepared baking sheet in neat rows, about ¼ inch apart. Do not discard the marinade. Place the baking sheet in the center of the preheated oven, and bake until crisped, about 15 to 17 minutes. The tofu may blacken a bit since the sugar in the honey will caramelize, but take care not to allow it to burn.

While the tofu is baking, return the remaining marinade to the saucepan, add the 2 tablespoons of cornstarch, and whisk to combine well. Return the saucepan to the stovetop and heat it over medium heat until the sauce thickens again, whisking constantly.

Serve the tofu over brown rice. Top with the sauce.

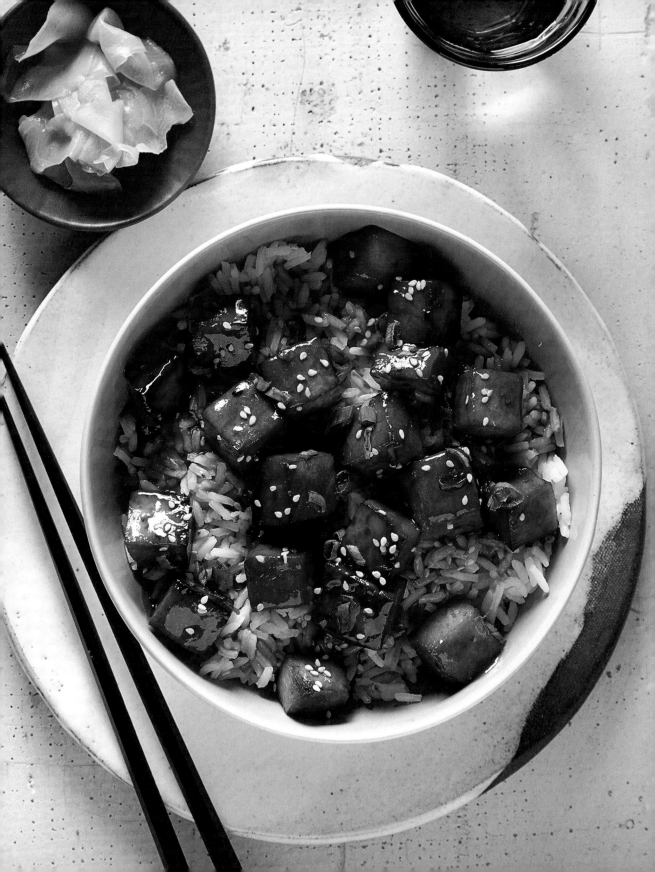

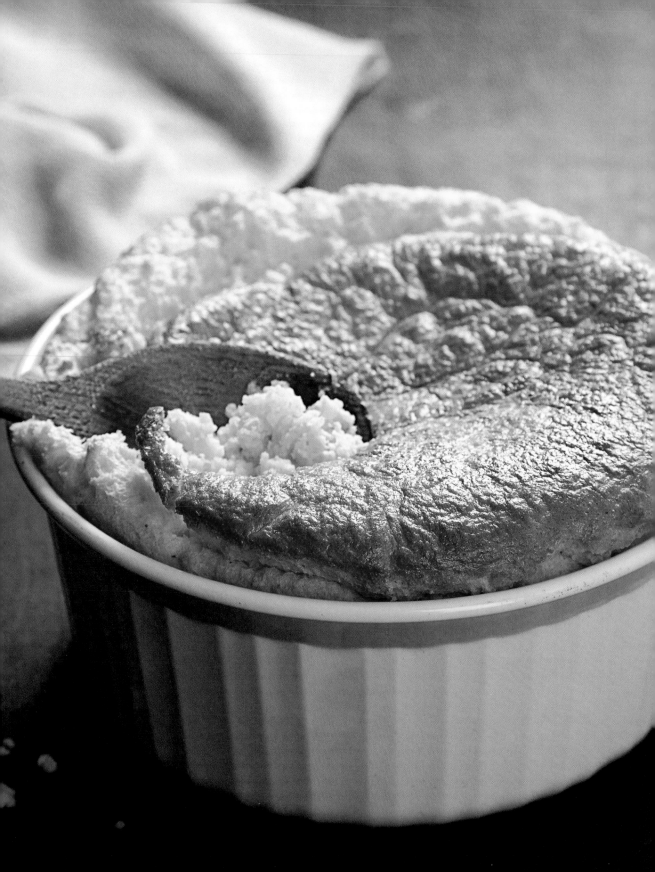

# CORNMEAL SPOONBREAD

*Makes* 4 servings

THIS SPOONBREAD IS SOMETHING LIKE A SOUFFLÉ, BUT I DON'T SEPARATE THE EGGS. I used to separate the eggs, whip up the whites with terrific effort, then gently fold them in. The dish was beautifully domed and fell a bit within 5 minutes of being taken out of the oven. Then one day, just like that, I stopped separating the eggs. If there was a difference in how puffy the final product was after 5 minutes of taking the dish out of the oven, I'll be a monkey's uncle. If you ever have occasion to make gluten-free cornmeal spoonbread for the queen of England, go the extra mile and separate the eggs.

2 cups (16 fluid ounces) milk

4 tablespoons (56 g) unsalted butter, at room temperature

½ teaspoon (3 g) kosher salt

1 cup (132 g) coarsely ground yellow cornmeal

4 eggs (200 g, weighed out of shell), at room temperature, lightly beaten

PREHEAT THE OVEN TO 375°F. GREASE A 6-INCH DIAMETER OVENPROOF CASSEROLE DISH WITH unsalted butter and set it aside.

In a medium saucepan, slowly heat the milk, butter, and salt until the mixture boils. Once it boils, turn down to a simmer, add the cornmeal, and cook, whisking constantly. It will suddenly come together. Set the mixture aside to cool for about 10 minutes.

Once the mixture has cooled, add the eggs, one at a time, whisking well after each addition, until smooth. Spoon the mixture into the prepared casserole dish, place it in the middle of the preheated oven, and bake for 1 hour, until browned on top.

Cut two small slits into the top of the spoonbread as soon as it comes out of the oven. This will allow some steam to escape and the casserole to remain puffy. Serve immediately.

# TOMATO POLENTA

*Makes* 4 servings

THIS IS SIMILAR TO THE BASIC POLENTA WE MAKE FOR POLENTA PIZZA (SEE PAGE 157), but it's jazzed up with tomatoes. Since the tomatoes add a bunch of moisture to the mixture, we use as much cornmeal as we do milk to keep everything in proper balance. This dish is warm and comforting and makes a beautiful base for some grilled chicken.

1 (28-ounce) can whole, peeled tomatoes

1 cup (8 fluid ounces) milk

1 teaspoon (6 g) kosher salt

1 cup (132 g) polenta cornmeal

2 ½ ounces Parmigiano-Reggiano cheese, finely grated, plus more for topping

REMOVE THE TOMATOES FROM THE CAN, CHOP THEM ROUGHLY, AND SET THEM ASIDE. IN A large saucepan, warm the milk over medium heat until simmering gently. You don't want it to boil. Add the chopped tomatoes with their juice, plus the salt, to the pan, and stir to combine. The acid in the tomatoes may cause the milk to begin to curdle, which is fine.

Continue to heat the milk mixture until it returns to simmering. Once the liquid is simmering, add the polenta cornmeal in a slow but steady stream, whisking constantly, making sure there are no lumps. Reduce the heat to low, and continue to whisk until the mixture thickens, about 5 to 7 minutes. Remove the pan from the heat and stir in the Parmigiano-Reggiano cheese until it is fully incorporated and melted. Serve with a few extra shavings of cheese.

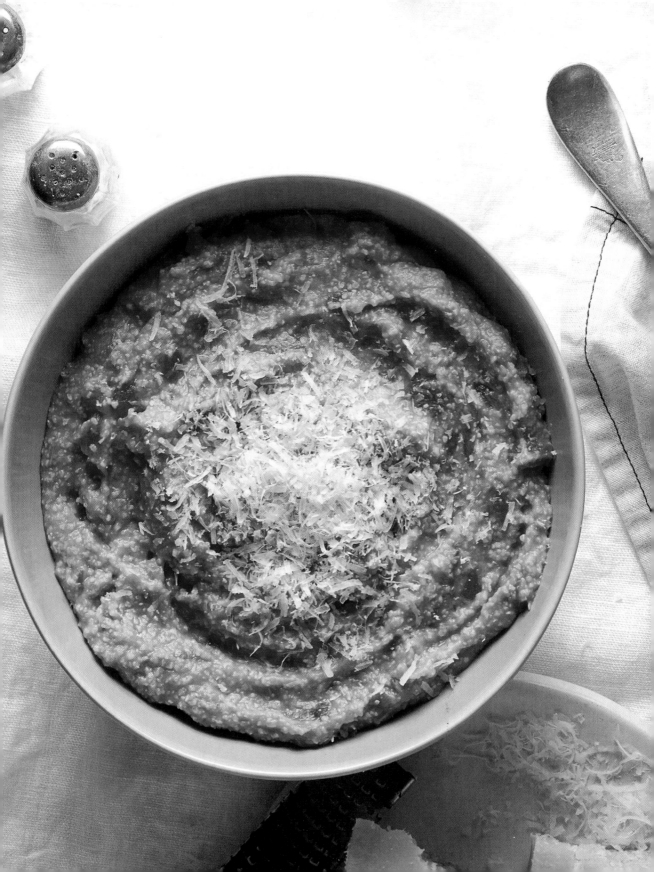

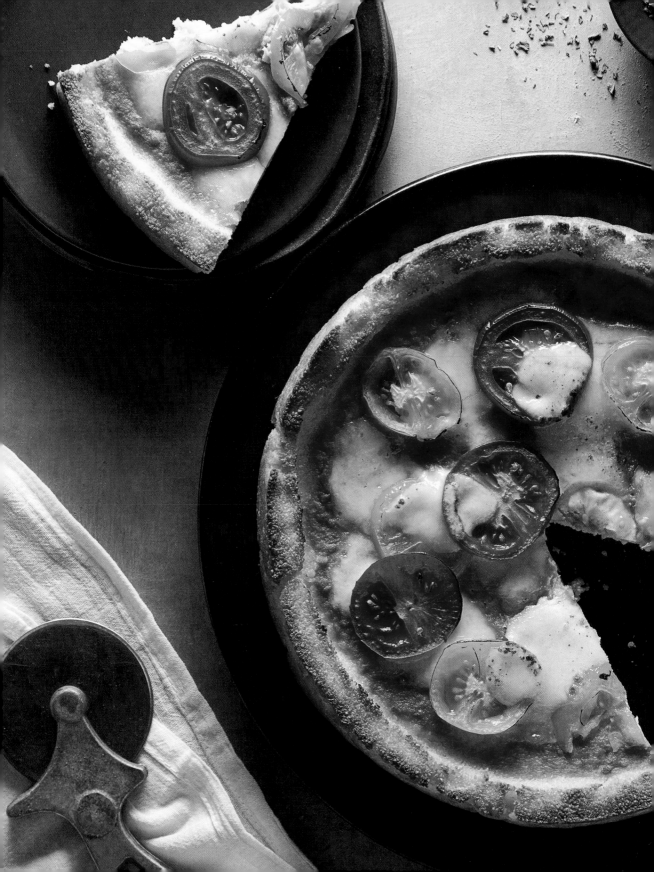

# POLENTA PIZZA

*Makes* 4 servings

I FEEL LIKE I'M CHEATING ON THIS ONE. IT'S REALLY MORE OF A CONCEPT THAN A RECIPE. The idea is that, for the purpose of staving off boredom (yours and that of your cooking audience), you make a quick batch of polenta, press it into the bottom of a springform pan, and make it into pizza by baking it with toppings of your choice. Then slice it into wedges and serve. If you are patient enough to wait for the polenta crust to brown, it will be a crispy delight that you can really sink your teeth into.

1¼ cups (10 fluid ounces) vegetable stock

1¼ cups (10 fluid ounces) milk

2 tablespoons (28 g) unsalted butter

1 teaspoon (6 g) kosher salt

1¼ cups (165 g) polenta cornmeal

2 to 3 tablespoons (28 to 42 g) extra-virgin olive oil, for brushing

Sauce and cheese toppings of your choosing

GREASE A 9-INCH SPRINGFORM PAN WITH UNSALTED BUTTER AND SET IT ASIDE. PREHEAT THE oven to 400°F.

In a medium saucepan, bring the stock, milk, butter, and salt to a boil over medium-high heat. Lower the heat to a simmer and add the polenta cornmeal, whisking constantly. It will come together suddenly. Remove the saucepan from the heat, and immediately spread the mixture on the bottom of the springform pan. With wet hands, push the polenta into the edges of the pan to create a raised edge. Brush the olive oil over the polenta crust. This will help it to brown in the oven.

Place the pan in the center of the preheated oven and bake for about 15 minutes, or until the crust is a bit browned. Remove it from the oven and top the polenta with some tomato sauce and some cheese, or whatever else you like, in whatever way you like. It can stand up to pretty much any topping.

Return the dish to the hot oven and bake for another 5 minutes, or until the cheese has melted. Allow the pizza to cool in the pan for approximately 5 minutes before popping off the sides of the springform pan and transferring the pizza to a flat surface. Slice the pie into 8 wedges with a large serrated knife. Serve immediately.

# ZUCCHINI PIZZA

*Makes* one 13-inch pizza

WE GROW ZUCCHINI AT HOME DURING THE SUMMERTIME. AS ANYONE WHO HAS ever done so knows, it is a prolific vegetable. It begs to be used quickly and efficiently, lest it take over your life. This zucchini pizza is not only an efficient use of zucchini, but it may be one of my favorite versions of pizza of all time, which includes actual bread-based pizza—with or without gluten. The addition of both mozzarella cheese and tapioca starch/flour to the dough makes for a pizza base that is both deeply flavorful and foldable. That's right. You can actually fold a slice of this pizza and enjoy it as you would thin crust 'za.

I squeeze the liquid out of grated zucchini by placing it, about 2 cups at a time, in a fine mesh bag (like a nut milk bag) or tea towel, closing the bag or rolling up the towel, and twisting it to squeeze out all of the liquid.

4 cups (440 g) grated fresh zucchini (from about 2 medium zucchini)

2 ounces Parmigiano-Reggiano cheese, finely grated

8 ounces low-moisture mozzarella cheese, grated

2 eggs (100 g, weighed out of shell), at room temperature, beaten

½ cup (80 g) tapioca starch/flour

Optional spices: 1 tablespoon dried oregano, 1½ teaspoons dried basil, ½ teaspoon garlic powder

Optional pizza toppings: tomato sauce, more mozzarella cheese, gluten-free pepperoni, sautéed mushrooms

PREHEAT THE OVEN TO 450°F. PLACE A PIZZA STONE OR OVERTURNED BAKING SHEET IN THE oven as it preheats. Line a pizza peel or other flat surface (like a large cutting board) with a sheet of unbleached parchment paper and set it aside.

In a large bowl, place the dry grated zucchini, Parmigiano-Reggiano cheese, mozzarella cheese, eggs, tapioca starch/flour, and optional spices. Mix to combine well. The mixture will be thick but soft. Transfer it to the parchment paper and, with a moistened silicone spatula or large spoon, spread it into a 13-inch round in one even layer. With wet hands or the side of the spatula or spoon, even the edges around the perimeter.

Slide the pizza on the parchment off the peel or cutting board onto the pizza stone or overturned baking sheet in the oven. Bake for 15 minutes or until the pizza is an even light golden-brown color on top. Remove from the oven, spread your desired pizza toppings on top, and return to the oven for another 5 minutes or until any cheese is melted and the edges are crisp. Remove the pizza from the oven and allow to set for 2 minutes before slicing into wedges and serving warm.

Any leftover pieces can be covered and refrigerated for at least 3 days and enjoyed cold or refreshed in a warm toaster oven or microwave before serving.

# NOODLE KUGEL

*Makes* 6 to 8 servings

I WISH I HAD A BETTER NAME FOR THIS, BUT "NOODLE PUDDING" DOESN'T QUITE FIT, SO we'll stick with Noodle Kugel. It's a decadent blend of noodles, eggs, butter, cream cheese, sour cream, and ricotta cheese, baked with a cereal topping. I suspect it's a dessert masquerading as food, so there are more than a few cheers when I treat my children to it.

1 pound (16 ounces) short, gluten-free dried pasta (elbows, penne, small shells, etc.)

8 tablespoons (112 g) unsalted butter, at room temperature

8 eggs (400 g, weighed out of the shell), separated into yolks and whites

½ cup plus 2 tablespoons (72 g) confectioners' sugar

1 (8-ounce) package cream cheese, at room temperature

1½ cups (384 g) sour cream

1 pound (16 ounces) low-moisture ricotta cheese

½ teaspoon (3 g) kosher salt

⅛ teaspoon cream of tartar

TOPPING

4 tablespoons unsalted butter, melted

⅔ cup crushed gluten-free corn flakes

PREHEAT THE OVEN TO 350°F. GREASE A 13 × 9-INCH BAKING DISH WITH UNSALTED BUTTER and set it aside.

In a large pot of boiling water, cook the pasta to an al dente texture, drain it, and return it to the hot pot. To the pasta, add the butter and stir to melt it and coat the pasta. Set the pot aside.

In a large bowl, place the egg yolks, sugar, cream cheese, sour cream, ricotta cheese, and salt, and beat until pale golden in color. In a separate bowl, beat the egg whites with the cream of tartar until stiff peaks form, and then carefully fold the egg whites into the egg yolk mixture with a wide spatula. Add the mixture to the pasta pot, and stir gently with the wide spatula to combine well, then scrape everything into the prepared baking dish, smoothing the top.

In a small bowl, combine the melted butter and crushed corn flakes and mix well. Sprinkle the topping over the pasta mixture in the baking dish as evenly as possible. Cover the baking dish completely with aluminum foil; place it in the center of the preheated oven and bake for 45 minutes. Then uncover the dish and bake for another 10 to 15 minutes or until lightly browned on top.

Cut the kugel into squares and serve warm or at room temperature.

# TOMATO SOUP

*Makes* about 6 cups soup

WITH ITS DEEP RED COLOR AND LUXURIOUS THICKNESS, THIS TOMATO SOUP IS more versatile and robust than you might otherwise imagine. It is deliciously simple served with a buttered dinner roll (see page 99) or some cheese crackers (see page 57), but it can also be a warm and filling meal when served the childhood classic way: with a quick grilled cheese.

1 (28-ounce) can whole, peeled tomatoes (preferably with basil)

1½ teaspoons (9 g) kosher salt

⅛ teaspoon freshly ground black pepper

4 tablespoons (56 g) extra-virgin olive oil

1 medium yellow onion, peeled and diced

3 garlic cloves, crushed whole and peeled

2 tablespoons dried oregano

2 tablespoons tomato paste

2 carrots, peeled and grated

2 large roasting potatoes, peeled and medium diced

2 cups (16 fluid ounces) vegetable stock

PREHEAT THE OVEN TO 375°F. LINE A RIMMED BAKING SHEET WITH ALUMINUM FOIL AND grease with cooking spray. Remove the tomatoes from the can and drain them (reserving the liquid). Ensure that all the tomatoes are peeled, slice them in half, and place them in a single layer on the prepared baking sheet. Sprinkle the tomatoes with ½ teaspoon of the salt and the pepper, then drizzle them evenly with 2 tablespoons olive oil. Place the baking sheet in the center of the preheated oven, and bake until the tomatoes begin to brown, about 20 to 25 minutes.

While the tomatoes are roasting, in a medium saucepan, heat the remaining 2 tablespoons of oil over medium-high heat. Add the onion and crushed whole garlic and cook until the onion is translucent and the garlic fragrant, about 6 minutes. Remove and discard the garlic. Crush or rub the dried oregano in your hands to release the herb's oils before adding it and the tomato paste to the saucepan. Stir to combine. Add the carrots, potatoes, vegetable stock, remaining 1 teaspoon of salt, and 2 cups (16 fluid ounces) of water, and continue to cook until the liquid is boiling. Turn the heat down to a simmer and cook until the carrots and potatoes are beginning to soften, about 10 minutes.

Add the roasted tomatoes and all of the roasting bits from the baking sheet to the saucepan, stir to combine, and return the soup to a simmer. Allow the soup to simmer gently, uncovered, until it thickens and the carrots and potatoes are very tender, about another 15 to 20 minutes.

For a smoother consistency, purée a portion of the soup with an immersion blender.

# CHEDDAR BROCCOLI SOUP

*Makes* about 6 cups soup

CHEDDAR BROCCOLI SOUP, WHEN MADE WELL, IS MOST CERTAINLY NOT CHEESE FONDUE with broccoli. This soup has the sharp flavor of Cheddar cheese and is easily eaten with a soupspoon. It begins with a roux made among sautéed aromatics. The milk, cream, and Cheddar cheese are added at the very end so that they don't have a chance to curdle in the hot liquid.

1 small bunch fresh broccoli

4 cups (32 fluid ounces) vegetable stock, divided

4 tablespoons (56 g) unsalted butter, chopped

1 small yellow onion, peeled and diced

2 garlic cloves, crushed whole and peeled

2 carrots, peeled and shredded

½ teaspoon (3 g) kosher salt

⅛ teaspoon freshly ground black pepper

¼ cup (35 g) Basic Gum-Free Gluten-Free Flour (see page 21)

2 dried bay leaves

1 cup milk (8 fluid ounces)

½ cup (4 fluid ounces) heavy whipping cream

8 ounces sharp yellow Cheddar cheese, grated

SEPARATE THE BROCCOLI FLORETS FROM THE STEMS, AND RINSE THEM CLEAN. IN A SMALL, heavy-bottom saucepan, place about 1 cup of stock and bring to a simmer over medium-high heat. Place the broccoli florets in the simmering stock and cook until just bright green (about 2 minutes). Remove the florets, place in a separate small bowl, and set aside. Remove the stock from the heat and set it aside.

In a large, heavy-bottom saucepan, place the butter and melt over medium heat. Add the onion, garlic, carrots, salt, and pepper, and mix to combine. Sauté the vegetables until the onion is translucent and the garlic is fragrant (about 6 minutes). Remove and discard the garlic. Add the gum-free flour blend, whisk to combine, and cook, whisking frequently, until the flour begins to smell nutty (about 2 minutes). Slowly add all of the stock (the 3 cups remaining, plus the cup used to blanch the broccoli), whisking constantly, until well combined. Add the bay leaves, bring to a simmer, and cook, stirring occasionally, until the mixture thickens (about 8 minutes).

Remove and discard the bay leaves, add the milk and cream, and continue to cook for another 2 minutes or until beginning to thicken. Add the Cheddar cheese, and cook until the cheese is melted. Serve immediately with the blanched broccoli florets.

I don't recommend freezing this soup, as milk-based soups tend to separate if frozen.

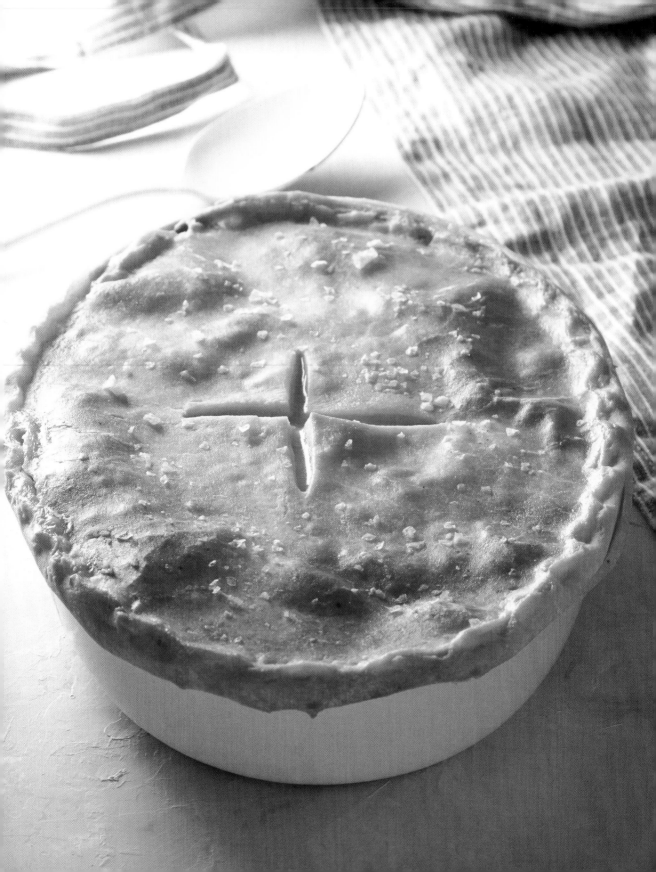

# COMFORTING DINNERS: JUST LIKE MOM USED *to* MAKE

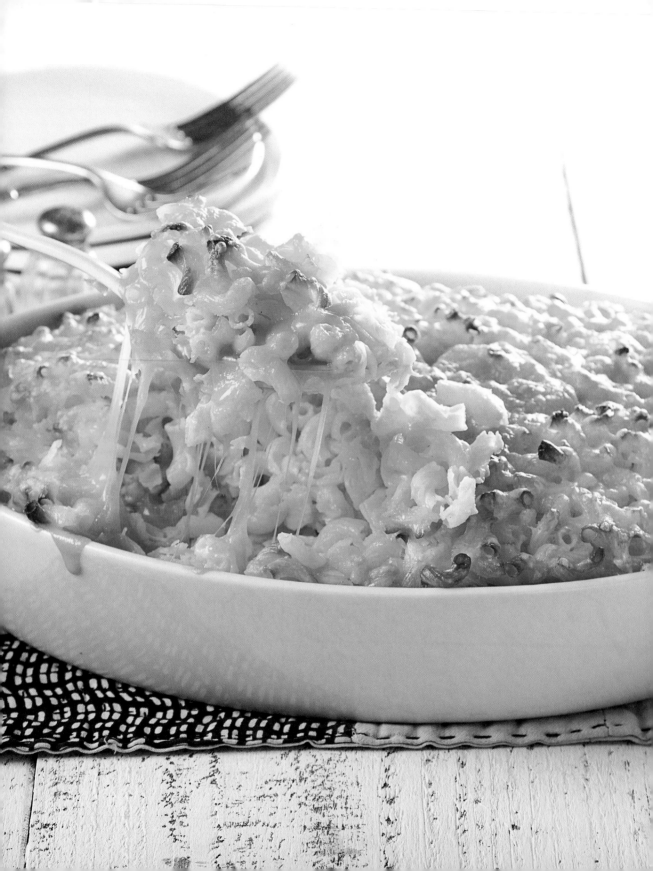

# MACARONI AND CHEESE

*Makes* 4 servings

THIS RECIPE FOR MACARONI AND CHEESE IS CASSEROLE-STYLE WITH EGGS, POURED into a 13 × 9-inch baking dish, covered, and baked until firm. Only one of my children will eat the stovetop version, and I have to assume it's a matter of texture. All three of them will eat it baked. This is also a great make-ahead dish. Just prepare the pasta mixture, pour it into a prepared baking dish, cover it tightly with foil and plastic wrap, and freeze it. When you are ready to serve it, there is no need to defrost it first. Just remove the plastic wrap but retain the foil, pop it in a preheated oven, and bake according to the recipe directions.

1 pound (16 ounces) short, gluten-free dried pasta (elbows, penne, small shells, etc.)

8 tablespoons (112 g) unsalted butter, at room temperature

4 eggs (200 g, weighed out of shell), at room temperature

1 can (12 fluid ounces) evaporated milk

1 teaspoon (6 g) kosher salt

Freshly ground black pepper, to taste

12 ounces Cheddar cheese, grated

PREHEAT THE OVEN TO 350°F, AND GREASE A 13 × 9-INCH BAKING DISH.

In a large pot of boiling water, cook the pasta to an al dente texture (shave a couple of minutes off the package directions). Drain the pasta and return it to the hot pot, off the stovetop.

Add the butter to the pot of cooked pasta and toss gently until the butter is entirely melted into the hot pasta. It should take you 2 minutes or less.

Beat the eggs in a separate, medium bowl. Add the milk, salt, and pepper, and whisk to combine. Add a few tablespoons of the hot pasta to the egg mixture. This will temper the eggs by slowly coaxing them up to a warmer temperature.

Add the egg mixture to the pasta pot, then the grated cheese, and stir gently to combine without breaking the pasta. Spread the entire mixture evenly into the prepared baking dish, cover the dish with foil, and bake in the preheated oven for about 25 minutes or until it is bubbling around the edges and the eggs are set. Uncover and bake for another 5 minutes until browned on top. Cool 10 minutes, and then slice into squares and serve.

*Shoestring* SAVINGS | ON A SHOESTRING: 27¢/ounce
ON THE SHELF: 87¢/ounce

COMFORTING DINNERS: JUST LIKE MOM USED TO MAKE

# APPLE-LEEK-SAUSAGE CORNBREAD STUFFING DINNER

*Makes* 6 servings

I HAD ALWAYS MADE THIS CORNBREAD STUFFING WITH APPLES AND LEEKS, BUT IT'S SO hearty and everyone in my family loves it so well that I started experimenting with adding some protein to make it a satisfying main dish. The sausage, removed from its casing and crumbled, does just the trick. And the old-fashioned cornbread helps to stretch the sausage, so it feeds more hungry people.

1½ pounds sweet sausage, casing removed

6 tablespoons (84 g) unsalted butter

3 leeks, cleaned, trimmed, and sliced thinly in cross-section

5 firm apples, peeled, cored, and diced (Granny Smith work well here)

2 tablespoons poultry seasoning

½ teaspoon (3 g) kosher salt

⅛ teaspoon freshly ground black pepper

3 tablespoons fresh parsley, chopped

1 recipe Old-Fashioned Cornbread (see page 97), crumbled

3 eggs (150 g, weighed out of shell), at room temperature, beaten

¼ cup (2 fluid ounces) milk

2 cups (16 fluid ounces) Chicken Stock (see page 26)

IN A MEDIUM SAUCEPAN OVER MEDIUM HEAT, COOK THE SAUSAGE UNTIL COOKED THROUGH and browned, about 5 minutes. It helps to break up the sausage into small pieces while it is cooking. The sausage cooks faster, and you can then better distribute it throughout the stuffing. Remove the sausage from the pan and set it aside to drain in a medium-size bowl.

In the same medium saucepan with the sausage drippings, melt the butter over very low heat. Once the butter is melted, add the leeks, apples, poultry seasoning, salt, pepper, and parsley, and cook, covered, over medium-low heat until the leeks and apples are soft and the flavors are married. The mixture should be very fragrant.

Add the crumbled cornbread to the mixture and stir to combine. Break up any very large pieces with your stirring spoon. Set the mixture aside to cool for about 10 to 15 minutes.

Preheat the oven to 375°F. Grease a 12 × 9-inch dish with unsalted butter and set it aside.

In a separate small bowl, place the eggs and milk and whisk to combine. Then add the chicken stock, and mix to combine. After the stuffing mixture has cooled off, temper the beaten egg mixture by adding a few spoonfuls of the stuffing mixture and stirring gently. This allows the eggs to get accustomed to the temperature of the warm stuffing mixture without being scrambled. Add the tempered egg mixture to the rest of the stuffing mixture, and stir gently until combined. Add the sausage to the mixture, and stir until the sausage is evenly distributed throughout.

Spread the mixture evenly in the greased baking dish and smooth the top. You don't want any big pieces of cornbread sticking up. They'll burn when you brown the stuffing.

Cover the dish completely with foil and place it in the preheated oven. Bake for 35 to 40 minutes or until the eggs are set. Uncover and bake for another 7 to 10 minutes, until the stuffing is nicely browned. Serve warm or at room temperature.

# MEATLOVE

*Makes* 6 servings

I F THERE IS A TRULY MEANINGFUL DIFFERENCE BETWEEN MEATLOAF AND MEATBALLS IN the home kitchen, it has thus far eluded me. I use one basic recipe for both shapes of this flavorful mixture of ground beef, breadcrumbs, cheese, eggs, milk, and spices. We call it Meatlove, since that is what my son thought it was called when he was rather small, and the name stuck. Who wants to eat something called "meatloaf" anyhow? It's descriptive, sure, but not exactly appetizing. Meatlove it is, then. And love it, we do.

½ cup (4 fluid ounces) milk

4 eggs (200 g, weighed out of shell)

1 cup (120 g) panko-style gluten-free breadcrumbs

2 ounces low-moisture mozzarella cheese, grated

½ ounce Parmigiano-Reggiano cheese, finely grated

2 tablespoons dried oregano (or 1 tablespoon chopped fresh oregano)

1 tablespoon dried basil (or 1½ teaspoons roughly chopped fresh basil)

1 tablespoon dried parsley (or 1½ teaspoons chopped fresh flat-leaf parsley)

2 garlic cloves, peeled and minced

½ teaspoon (3 g) kosher salt

⅛ teaspoon freshly ground black pepper

2 pounds 90% lean ground beef

2 to 4 cups Easy Homemade Tomato Sauce (optional) (see page 48)

¼ to ½ cup (56 to 112 g) extra-virgin olive oil (optional)

IN A LARGE BOWL, PLACE THE MILK AND EGGS, AND BEAT TO COMBINE. ADD THE BREADCRUMBS, cheeses, oregano, basil, parsley, garlic, salt, and pepper, and mix to combine. Add the meat to the large bowl and, with clean hands, gently mix all the ingredients together.

If you are making meatballs, grease an oven-safe dish with at least 2-inch-high sides and pre-heat the oven to 350°F.

Divide the beef mixture into portions and shape into round meatballs about 1 inch in diame-ter. Place the meatballs at least 1 inch apart from one another in the baking dish, and cover with the optional tomato sauce or drizzle with olive oil. Place in the center of the preheated oven and bake for approximately 35 minutes, until cooked through.

If you are making meatloaf (or Meatlove): line a rimmed baking sheet with unbleached parch-ment paper, and preheat the oven to 350°F. Place the beef mixture onto the prepared baking sheet and shape into a loaf, place in the center of the oven, and bake for 45 to 60 minutes, until cooked through. If the top begins to brown before the meatloaf is cooked all the way through, tent it with a piece of foil and finish baking. Cut into ½ to ¾ inch thick slices to serve.

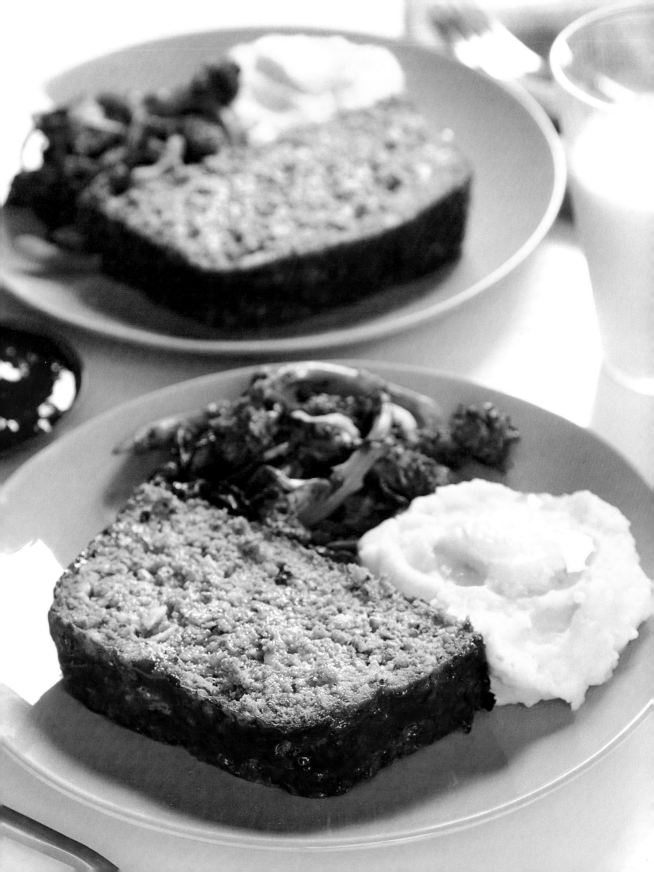

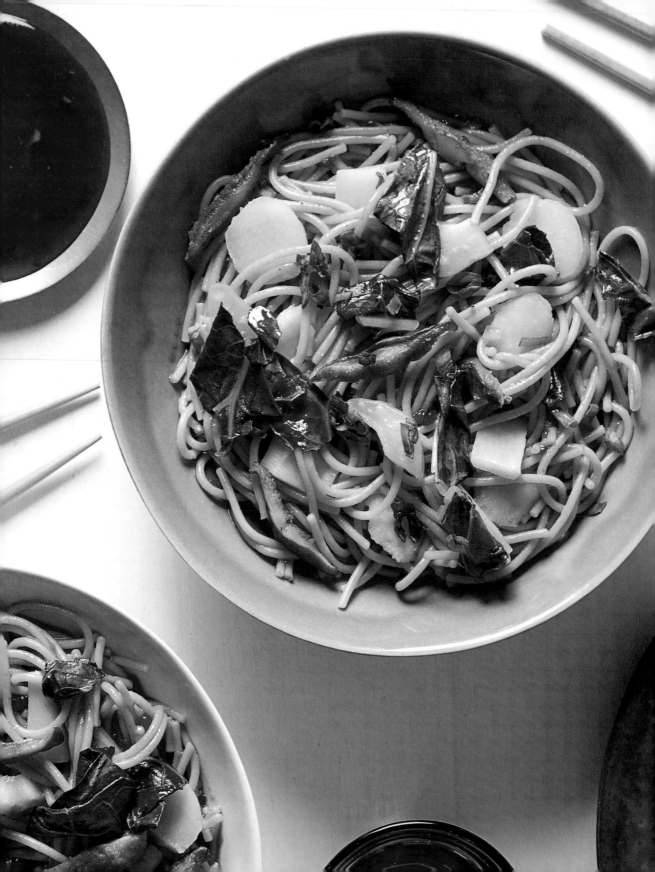

# LO MEIN

*Makes* 4 to 5 servings

THERE ARE A FEW CHINESE RESTAURANTS NEAR MY HOME THAT SERVE GLUTEN-FREE food. Although it's wonderful to have as an option, and I'm appreciative, we almost never go. When we're craving Chinese food, I usually would just rather make my own. With the money we'd spend on going to a restaurant, I can make dinner and dessert for a few nights straight. This recipe has just the right balance of spices and sweetness. I usually serve it with Szechuan Meatballs (see page 172) and Hoisin Sauce (see page 47).

2 garlic cloves, peeled and minced

2 tablespoons (28 g) toasted sesame oil

3½ cups (28 fluid ounces) Chicken Stock (see page 26)

½ teaspoon freshly ground black pepper

2 tablespoons (42 g) honey

2 tablespoons (27 g) packed light-brown sugar

2 tablespoons (42 g) unsulfured molasses

2 tablespoons rice vinegar

½ cup gluten-free soy sauce or tamari

2 tablespoons (18 g) cornstarch

1 pound (16 ounces) dried gluten-free spaghetti

IN A MEDIUM SAUCEPAN, SAUTÉ THE GARLIC IN SESAME OIL UNTIL FRAGRANT (ABOUT 2 TO 3 minutes). Add the chicken stock, pepper, honey, brown sugar, molasses, vinegar, soy sauce, and cornstarch to the saucepan. Whisk until the ingredients are well combined. Bring to a boil, then lower the heat to medium high and simmer gently for 8 to 10 minutes or until the mixture is reduced by nearly half and is thickened.

While the sauce is reducing, boil a large pot of water. To the boiling water, add the spaghetti and cook to an al dente texture. Drain the spaghetti, rinse it with cold water, drain it again, and place it in a large serving bowl. Pour the thickened sauce over the spaghetti and toss it with tongs to coat. Serve immediately.

COMFORTING DINNERS: JUST LIKE MOM USED TO MAKE

# SZECHUAN MEATBALLS

*Makes* about 18 meatballs

THE SECRET TO FLAVORFUL SZECHUAN MEATBALLS IS TO ALLOW THE GROUND BEEF TO marinate so it absorbs all the flavors in the soy sauce, honey, vinegar, and ginger. Be sure to use ground beef that is at least 90 percent lean. If you use beef that is less lean, the fat drains onto the pan when the meatballs are baked, and much of the flavor drains right along with it. Pity. The sesame oil in the marinade is much tastier and less greasy than the fat in the ground beef. I usually serve these meatballs with Lo Mein (see page 168) and Hoisin Sauce (see page 47).

¼ cup gluten-free soy sauce or tamari

2 tablespoons (42 g) honey

⅛ teaspoon freshly ground black pepper

¼ cup rice vinegar

¼ cup (56 g) toasted sesame oil

2 tablespoons fresh ginger, minced

2 tablespoons (18 g) cornstarch

2 eggs (100 g, weighed out of shell), at room temperature, beaten

1½ teaspoons Chinese-Style Hot Sauce (optional) (see page 46)

1½ pounds 90% lean ground beef

PREHEAT THE OVEN TO 375°F.

In a large bowl, whisk together the soy sauce, honey, pepper, vinegar, sesame oil, ginger, cornstarch, eggs, and optional hot sauce, until well combined.

Add the ground beef to the bowl. With clean hands (or a large fork), mix gently to combine the sauce with the ground beef. After mixing, allow the beef to absorb the other ingredients by covering the bowl and letting it sit at room temperature for 10 to 15 minutes.

Divide the meat mixture and roll into balls 1½ inches in diameter. Arrange 1 inch apart on lined rimmed baking sheets.

Bake in the preheated oven for 20 to 25 minutes or until nicely browned and cooked through. Serve immediately.

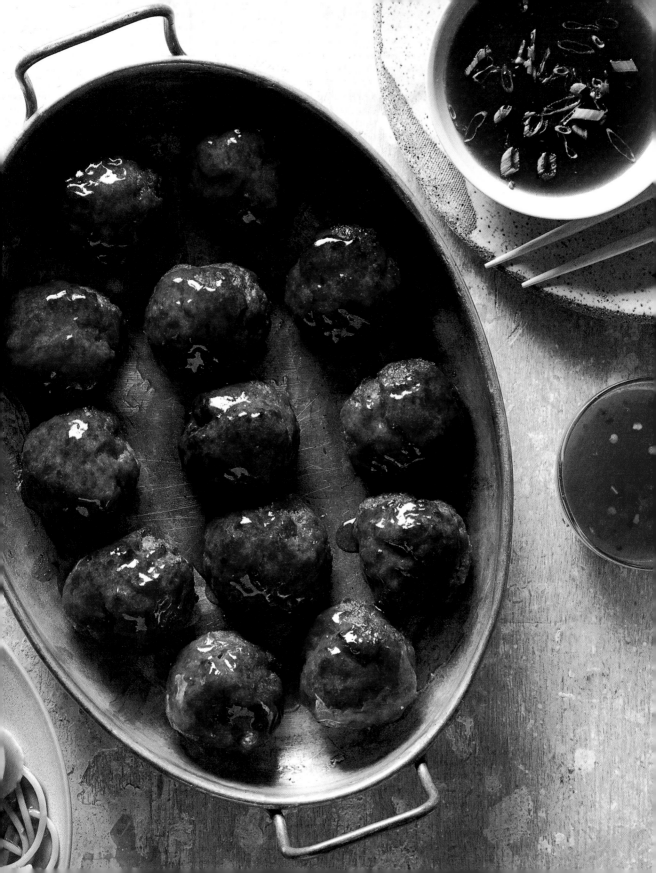

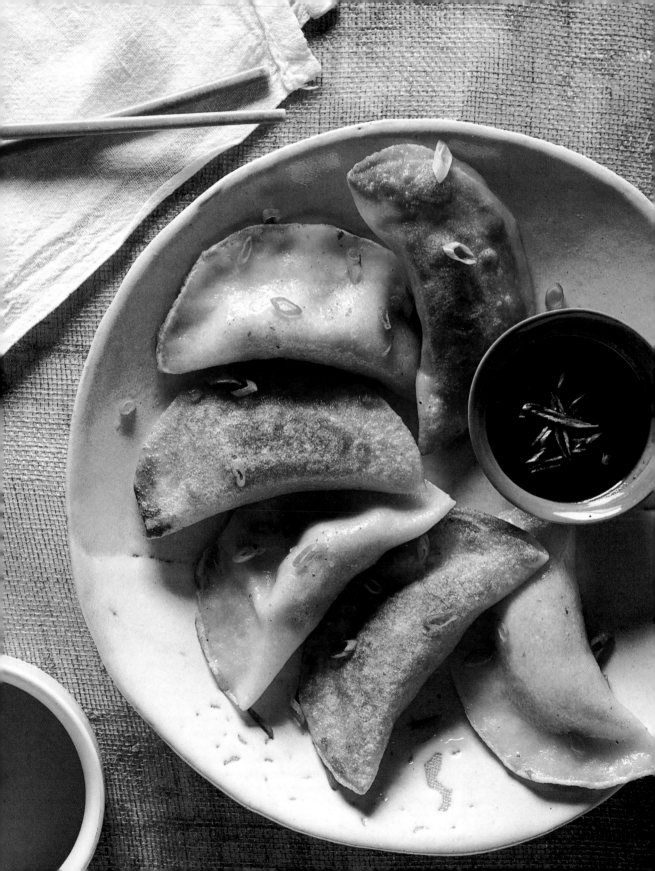

# BEEF POTSTICKERS

*Makes* 4 servings

I WON'T LIE TO YOU: I DON'T USUALLY FRY THESE. THEY'RE DELICIOUS FRIED, BUT THEY'RE just enough work as it is. To me, eating them as is strikes the right balance between effort and enjoyment. If you're craving fried potstickers, though, shallow fry these after they're boiled. And then be a good friend and send some to me.

| | |
|---|---|
| ¼ cup gluten-free soy sauce or tamari | 2 tablespoons fresh ginger, minced |
| 1 tablespoon (21 g) honey | 2 tablespoons (18 g) cornstarch |
| ⅛ teaspoon freshly ground black pepper | 1½ pounds 90% lean ground beef |
| ¼ cup rice vinegar | 15 to 20 Wonton Wrappers (see page 38), shaped into rounds |

IN A LARGE BOWL, WHISK TOGETHER THE SOY SAUCE, HONEY, PEPPER, VINEGAR, GINGER, AND cornstarch until well combined.

Add the ground beef to the bowl. With clean hands (or a large fork), mix gently to combine the sauce with the ground beef. After mixing, allow the beef to absorb the other ingredients by covering the bowl and letting it sit at room temperature for 10 to 15 minutes.

With wet hands, pinch off a portion of ground beef that is approximately ¾ inch in diameter and place it in the center of one wonton wrapper, leaving a border of at least 1 inch all around the wrapper. Again with wet hands, moisten the border of the wonton wrapper and fold it over, then press the edges together to seal it closed. Repeat the process with the remaining wonton wrappers.

Heat a large pot of boiling water, salt it liberally as it begins to boil, and gently drop the dumplings in the boiling water one at a time, in batches, so the pot is never too crowded, until cooked through, about 5 to 7 minutes. Carefully remove the dumplings from the water and serve hot or warm, with Hoisin Sauce (see page 47).

The filled dumplings can be wrapped tightly and frozen raw and then boiled from frozen, adding a minute or so to the boiling time.

*Shoestring* SAVINGS | ON A SHOESTRING: 33¢/potsticker
ON THE SHELF: $1.00/potsticker

COMFORTING DINNERS: JUST LIKE MOM USED TO MAKE

# SWEET AND SOUR CHICKEN

*Makes* 6 to 8 servings

WHEN BONELESS, SKINLESS CHICKEN BREAST IS ON SALE, I BUY LOTS OF IT, CLEAN it up, cut some into strips, some into chunks, divide the meat into groups of four to five portions, and freeze each portion in a separate, freezer-safe plastic storage bag. When I am ready to use a portion, I defrost it in the refrigerator overnight. I am always experimenting with different chicken dishes that are interesting and tasty without being fried. This sweet and sour chicken tastes remarkably like takeout, without the price tag and without the MSG.

2 pounds boneless, skinless chicken breast, cut into bite-size chunks (about 1 ½ inch square)

2 tablespoons gluten-free soy sauce or tamari

2 tablespoons (18 g) cornstarch

¼ teaspoon freshly ground black pepper

3 tablespoons (42 g) toasted sesame or neutral cooking oil

5 garlic cloves, crushed and peeled

2 carrots, peeled and cut into 1 ½-inch chunks

2 sweet bell peppers (any color), seeded and cut into 1 ½-inch chunks

4 scallions, trimmed and chopped in cross-section

1 recipe Sweet and Sour Sauce, at room temperature (see page 46)

IN A LARGE BOWL, TOSS THE CHICKEN, SOY SAUCE, CORNSTARCH, AND PEPPER UNTIL ALL THE pieces of chicken are coated. In a large nonstick skillet over medium-high heat, heat the oil and simmer the crushed garlic for 2 to 3 minutes, until it is fragrant and beginning to soften. Add the chicken to the pan and cook, in two batches if necessary, depending upon the size of the skillet, for 5 to 7 minutes or until lightly browned and cooked through. Remove the chicken from the pan, draining and leaving behind in the pan as much liquid as possible, and set it aside in a separate medium-size bowl.

Add the carrots and peppers to the pan and cook over medium-high heat in the liquid until softened, 4 to 5 minutes. Lower the heat and return the chicken mixture to the pan. Add the scallions and the Sweet and Sour Sauce to the pan and cook over low heat for 2 to 3 minutes, until the ingredients are well combined and the sauce is heated through. Serve immediately over cooked rice.

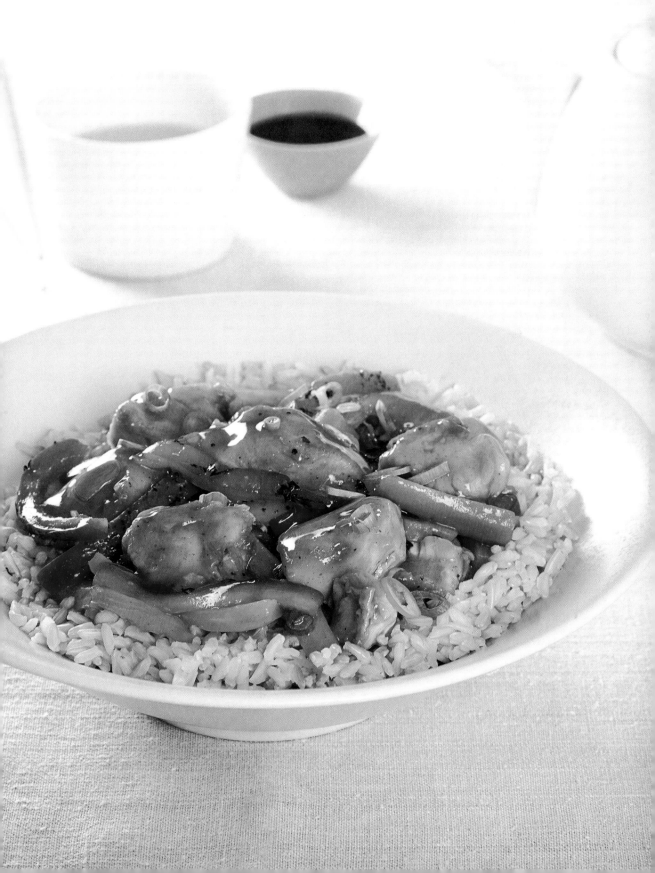

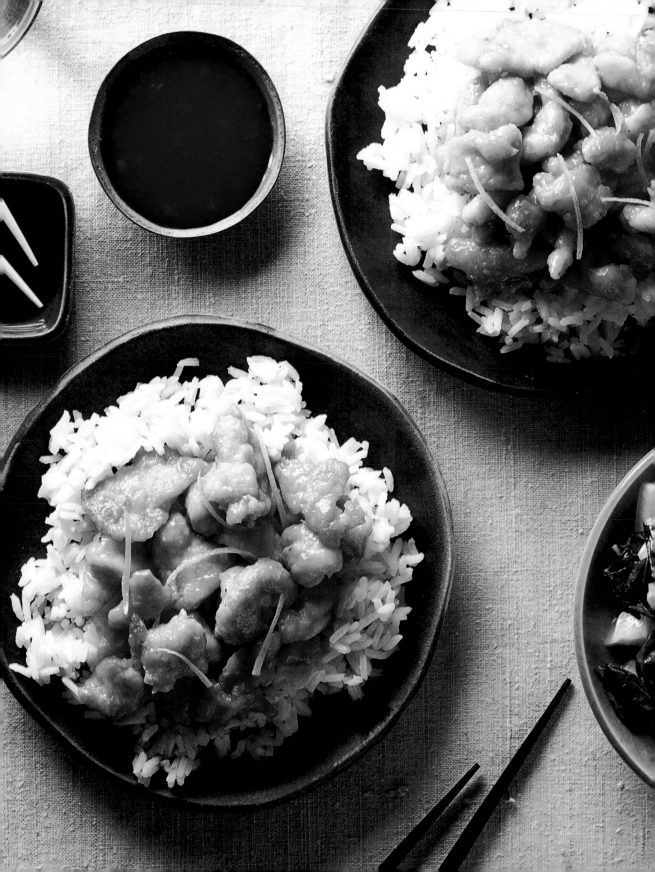

# LEMON CHICKEN, CHINESE-STYLE

*Makes* 4 servings

YOU DO NOT NEED A WOK TO MAKE THIS DISH. IT'S NICE TO USE ONE, SINCE THE FOOD cooks a bit quicker and a wok requires less oil than shallow frying, but at the end of the day, it's unnecessary. This really does taste authentic, and frying the chicken in small pieces like this and serving it over rice helps stretch the chicken while leaving your dinner companions satisfied and content.

2 cups (16 fluid ounces) Chicken Stock (see page 26)

Juice of 4 lemons

Finely grated zest of 1 lemon

¾ cup gluten-free soy sauce or tamari

3 tablespoons (40 g) packed light-brown sugar

3 eggs (150 g, weighed out of shell), at room temperature

¾ cup (108 g) cornstarch (or more, as needed)

1 pound boneless, skinless chicken breast, cut into small pieces (or strips)

¼ cup (56 g) neutral oil, for frying (more if frying in a shallow pan)

3 to 4 garlic cloves, peeled and minced

2 teaspoons ginger, minced (optional)

IN A MEDIUM-SIZE BOWL, WHISK TOGETHER THE CHICKEN STOCK, LEMON JUICE, LEMON ZEST, soy sauce, and brown sugar. Set it aside.

In a large bowl, beat the eggs with a couple of tablespoons of water. Place the cornstarch in a shallow dish. Dredge the chicken through the egg wash, allowing any excess to drop off. Place each piece in the cornstarch to coat lightly, shaking off any excess.

In a wok (or a large sauté pan, with more oil to shallow fry), heat the oil over medium-high heat. Add the chicken and fry until crisp, 2 to 3 minutes total, turning once. Remove the chicken and drain on paper towels. Repeat in batches if necessary, and add more oil as needed.

Add the soy sauce mixture to the pan with the garlic and the optional ginger, and bring to a boil. Return the chicken to the pan and stir-fry to warm, turning over to coat with the sauce. Serve immediately over cooked rice.

# ASIAN PORK LOIN

*Makes* 4 servings

THIS RECIPE MAKES ENOUGH MARINADE TO COOK A VEGETABLE, LIKE CHOPPED CARROTS or shredded cabbage, in the roasting pan with the pork. The meat will be so soft and moist, you can even shred it if you like. I like to buy a large, 4-pound pork loin when it is on sale, slice it in half, and marinate each of the 2 pounds according to this recipe in separate plastic bags (doubling the marinade). Once the meat has finished marinating, freeze one of the 2-pound packages, marinade and all. When you are ready to use the frozen and prepared pork loin, allow it to defrost in the refrigerator overnight, and then roast it according to the recipe directions. You'll be so glad you did.

½ cup gluten-free soy sauce or tamari

½ cup (112 g) toasted sesame or neutral oil

3 tablespoons gluten-free Worcestershire sauce

⅓ cup (73 g) packed light-brown sugar

2 tablespoons (42 g) unsulfured molasses

1 teaspoon black peppercorns (or 1½ teaspoons freshly ground black pepper)

3 tablespoons fresh ginger, minced

¼ cup rice vinegar

¼ cup balsamic vinegar

2 leeks, cleaned, trimmed, and sliced thinly in cross-section

4 garlic cloves, crushed and peeled

2 pounds pork loin, trimmed of the largest pieces of fat

IN A LARGE BOWL, PREPARE THE MARINADE BY WHISKING THE SOY SAUCE, OIL, WORCESTERSHIRE sauce, brown sugar, molasses, pepper, ginger, vinegars, leeks, and garlic until well combined.

Place the trimmed pork loin into a large, resealable plastic bag, pour the marinade into the bag on top of the meat, and seal the bag securely. With the bag sealed, gently massage the contents until the marinade has covered the meat completely. Place the bag, seam-side up, in a large bowl, and place the bowl in the refrigerator.

Allow the meat to marinate for at least 2 hours, and then turn the bag over so the other side of the meat is sitting in the marinade. Keep in the refrigerator for at least another 4 hours, or overnight.

Once the meat has finished marinating, preheat the oven to 325°F. Place the meat and the marinade in a roasting pan and place in the center of the preheated oven; cook for approximately 90 minutes or until the center of the roast reaches 160°F. Remove from the oven and allow the meat to rest for at least 10 to 15 minutes before slicing against the grain and serving.

# CHICKEN POTPIE

*Makes* 4 servings

TRADITIONAL CHICKEN POTPIES LIKE THIS ONE ARE SIMPLE TO PUT TOGETHER BUT somehow make a dramatic presentation for guests when you divide the recipe into personal-size pies. They smell like heaven and taste even better, especially when you get a perfect spoonful with just the right balance of buttery, flaky pastry crust and creamy, warm, and satisfying chicken and vegetable filling. And they can be assembled completely, then frozen for up to a month before baking.

½ recipe Savory Pastry Crust, chilled (see page 32)

3 tablespoons (42 g) extra-virgin olive oil

8 tablespoons (112 g) unsalted butter

3 large yellow onions, peeled and chopped

1½ pounds boneless, skinless chicken breasts

½ cup (70 g) Basic Gum-Free Gluten-Free Flour (see page 21)

4 to 6 cups (32 to 48 fluid ounces) Chicken Stock (see page 26)

¼ cup (2 fluid ounces) milk

½ teaspoon (3 g) kosher salt

⅛ teaspoon freshly ground black pepper

1 12-ounce package frozen mixed vegetables, thawed

Egg wash (1 egg plus 1 tablespoon water, beaten)

PREHEAT THE OVEN TO 375°F. GREASE A ROUND OVENPROOF BAKING DISH, AT LEAST 10 INCHES in diameter, with unsalted butter. Set the dish aside.

Press the pastry dough into a disk and place it on a lightly floured piece of unbleached parchment paper. Sprinkle it lightly with more flour, and roll out the dough until it is about ⅛ inch thick. Place the rolled-out dough, still on the parchment, in the refrigerator to chill.

In the meantime, make the filling. In a large saucepan, place the oil and 4 tablespoons of the butter and melt the butter over medium-high heat. Add the onions and sauté until translucent but not browned, about 6 minutes. Slice the chicken into a large dice, with pieces about 1 inch square, and place the chicken in the saucepan. Cook, stirring occasionally, until browned all over, about 4 minutes. Remove the chicken and onions from the pan and set them aside.

Add the remaining 4 tablespoons of butter, and melt it in the pan. Reduce the heat to low and add the gum-free flour, stirring constantly, until the flour is well incorporated and the mixture begins to smell a bit nutty (about 2 minutes). Add the chicken stock, milk, salt, and pepper, and stir to combine. Raise the heat to medium high once again, and cook until the mixture simmers and begins to thicken.

Once the mixture is simmering, add the thawed mixed vegetables and the cooked onion and chicken. Stir the mixture until all the ingredients are well combined. Pour the filling into the prepared baking dish. If making personal potpies, divide the filling among 4 oven-safe baking dishes, approximately 6 inches in diameter each.

Remove the pastry dough from the refrigerator. Turn the dough over, and place it on top of the filling in the baking dish. Gently remove the sheet of parchment paper from the top of the pie. Crimp the dough all around the perimeter of the pie, pressing it together with your fingers to seal it. With a very sharp knife, carefully cut an X in the middle of the pie to allow steam to escape during baking. With a pastry brush, paint the top of the pie with the egg wash. Again, if you are making four separate personal potpies, divide the dough evenly among the tops of the baking dishes in a similar manner to that described above.

Place the baking dish (or the 4 individual dishes) on a rimmed baking sheet, and place in the preheated oven and bake for about 35 minutes, until the top is lightly golden all over and the filling is bubbling. Serve immediately.

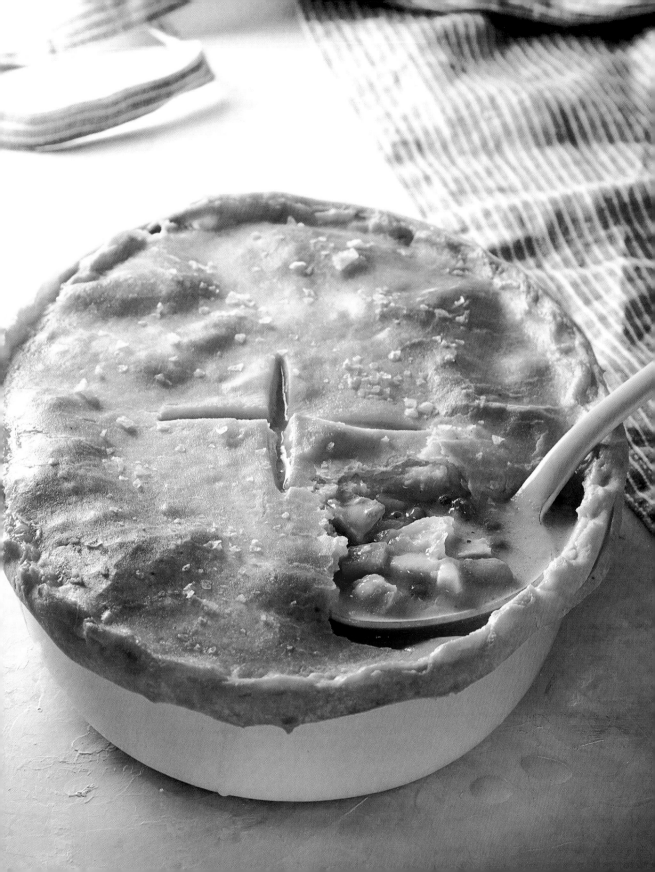

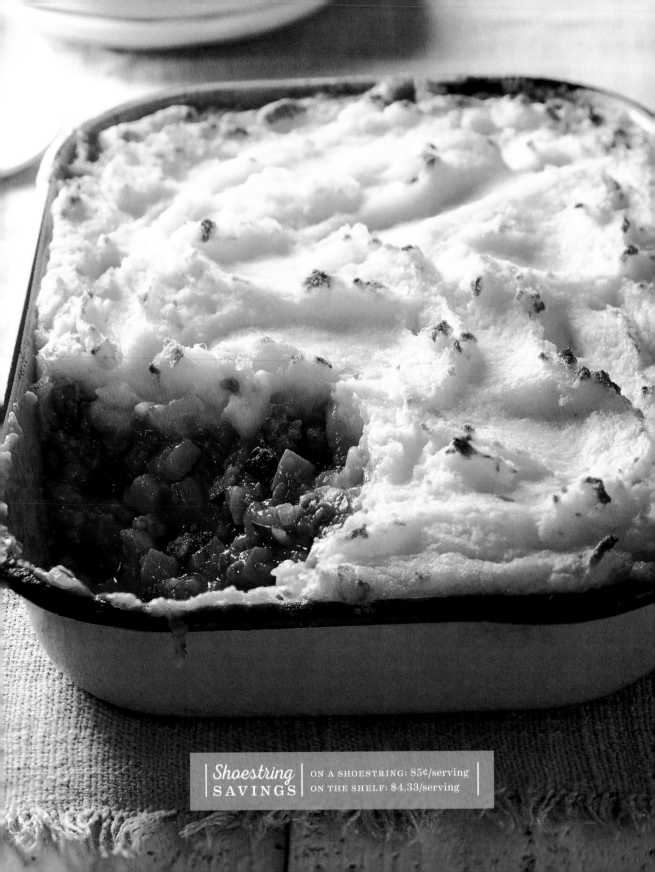

*Shoestring* SAVINGS | ON A SHOESTRING: 85¢/serving | ON THE SHELF: $4.33/serving

# SHEPHERD'S PIE

*Makes* 4 to 6 servings

SHEPHERD'S PIE IS ONE OF THOSE CLASSIC COMFORT FOODS THAT NEVER DISAPPOINTS. The essential elements are the browned ground beef, some vegetables, spices, and a mashed potato topping, so feel free to play with the types of vegetables and the types of potatoes that you use. I always use zucchini since it is so tasty with tomato sauce and adds nice moisture, and I prefer a mixture of red and sweet potatoes to make a colorful and savory crust. If you're feeling very generous, instead of the mashed potato crust, top the pie with rounds of raw Sweet Potato Biscuits (see page 107), and bake as usual or until the biscuits are nicely browned.

2 tablespoons (28 g) extra-virgin olive oil

1 large onion, peeled and diced

1 to 2 large carrots, peeled and shredded

1 large zucchini, chopped

1 pound 90% lean ground beef

2 tablespoons (18 g) Basic Gum-Free Gluten-Free Flour (see page 21)

1 cup (8 fluid ounces) Chicken Stock (see page 26)

3 tablespoons tomato paste

2 tablespoons gluten-free Worcestershire sauce

3 tablespoons chopped fresh parsley (or 1½ tablespoons dried)

2 pounds potatoes (a mixture of red and sweet, or either one alone), peeled

3 tablespoons (42 g) unsalted butter

½ cup (4 fluid ounces) milk

¼ teaspoon kosher salt, or to taste

PREHEAT THE OVEN TO 375°F. GREASE A 12 × 9 × 2-INCH BAKING DISH WITH UNSALTED BUTTER and set it aside.

In a large pan, heat the oil over medium-high heat. Add the onion, carrots, and zucchini, and cook until all the vegetables are soft and the onion and zucchini are translucent, about 7 minutes. Add the ground beef and cook until browned, another 5 minutes. Add the flour, and mix until well combined. Continue to cook for another minute, stirring frequently. Add the chicken stock, tomato paste, Worcestershire sauce, and parsley, and simmer uncovered until the mixture thickens, about 10 minutes. Spoon the beef mixture into the prepared baking dish, and set it aside.

In a medium to large pot, boil the potatoes in salted water, then reduce to a simmer and cook partly covered until the potatoes are fork-tender, about 20 minutes. Drain the water from the potatoes and mash them with a masher or fork, or pass them through a potato ricer or food mill. Add the butter and milk to the potatoes and salt to taste. Spread the mashed potatoes over the beef mixture. Make a crosshatch pattern over the top with a fork.

Bake in the center of the preheated oven for about 30 minutes. Move the dish up to the top of the oven and turn on the broiler for the last few minutes to crisp the potato crust. Serve immediately.

# BEEF POTPIE

*Makes* 6 servings

THIS DISH IS SIMILAR TO BEEF LASAGNA, BUT SINCE THE PASTA STARTS OUT DRY AND boils in chicken stock in the oven, it's richer and more satisfying (and significantly less time consuming to make). Add some bite-size broccoli crowns to the sour cream and ricotta mixture and you have a complete meal.

1 medium onion, peeled and chopped

2 tablespoons (28 g) extra-virgin olive oil

2 garlic cloves, peeled and minced

1½ pounds 90% lean ground beef

½ teaspoon (3 g) kosher salt

⅛ teaspoon freshly ground black pepper

3 cups Easy Homemade Tomato Sauce (see page 48)

1 cup (256 g) sour cream

8 ounces low-moisture ricotta cheese

1 pound (16 ounces) short, gluten-free dried pasta (elbows, penne, small shells, etc.)

2 cups (16 fluid ounces) Chicken Stock (see page 26)

8 ounces low-moisture mozzarella cheese, grated

1 recipe Pizza Dough, chilled (see page 36)

PREHEAT THE OVEN TO 375°F. GREASE A 13 × 9-INCH BAKING DISH WITH UNSALTED BUTTER and set it aside.

In a medium skillet over medium-high heat, sauté the chopped onion in the oil until the onion is translucent, about 6 minutes. Add the garlic to the pan, and sauté until fragrant, about 2 minutes. Add the ground beef, and cook until the beef is browned and cooked all the way through. Season with salt and pepper. Add 1½ cups of the tomato sauce to the beef mixture, stir to combine, and set the mixture aside.

In a medium-size bowl, place the sour cream and ricotta cheese, and mix until well combined.

Spoon the remaining 1½ cups of tomato sauce evenly over the bottom of the prepared baking dish. Sprinkle the dry pasta over the top of the tomato sauce, and then pour the 2 cups of chicken stock over the pasta. Spread the sour cream and ricotta cheese mixture, and then top with the beef mixture, each in a single layer across the pan. Sprinkle the mozzarella cheese evenly across the top.

Cover the baking dish tightly with foil and bake in the preheated oven for 30 to 35 minutes. Roll the pizza dough between two sheets of parchment into a 15 × 12-inch rectangle.

After the first 30 to 35 minutes of baking, remove the baking dish from the oven and remove the foil. Place the pizza dough on top of the baking dish, and carefully secure around the edges (the dish will be quite hot). Return the dish to the oven and bake 7 to 10 minutes more, until the dough is lightly browned on top. Allow to cool at least 15 minutes before serving.

# CHICKEN EN CROUTE

*Makes* 4 servings

I DON'T MAKE CHICKEN EN CROUTE TOO OFTEN BECAUSE I FEAR THAT AFTERWARD MY children will refuse all chicken served without cheese and preserves and uncloaked in pastry. It's kind of like sleeping in a tent in the desert and thinking it's a fine life until you sleep on clean, fresh sheets. You can't go back. Try this mix of sweet and savory, wrapped in flaky and buttery pastry, and I doubt you'll go back either.

1½ pounds boneless, skinless chicken breasts

½ teaspoon (3 g) kosher salt

⅛ teaspoon freshly ground black pepper

¼ cup fresh parsley, chopped (or 2 tablespoons dried parsley)

2 tablespoons (28 g) extra-virgin olive oil

1 recipe Savory Pastry Crust, chilled (see page 32)

4 ounces low-moisture mozzarella cheese, grated

½ cup apricot preserves

Egg wash (1 egg plus 1 tablespoon water, beaten)

PREHEAT THE OVEN TO 400°F. LINE BAKING SHEETS WITH UNBLEACHED PARCHMENT PAPER and set them aside.

Slice the chicken into a large dice, with pieces about 1 inch square, and season them with salt, pepper, and parsley. In a medium-size skillet, heat the oil over medium-high heat. Brown the chicken all over, for about 4 minutes total. Remove the chicken from the heat and set it aside.

Remove the pastry dough from the refrigerator and divide it into two equal portions. Place each on a separate lightly floured sheet of unbleached parchment paper, sprinkle lightly with more flour, and roll into a rectangle a bit more than ⅛ inch thick. Slice the dough into 4 rectangles, each approximately 6 × 3 inches. Lightly flour the rectangles of dough to prevent sticking, stack them on top of one another, and place in the refrigerator to chill until firm.

On one-half of each rectangle of dough, place about one-quarter of the chicken, then top with cheese and a spoonful of preserves. Fold over and pinch to secure the edges.

Transfer the pastries to the prepared baking sheets. Brush the egg wash over the top and seams of each pastry. This will help keep the pastries from opening and help them brown in the oven.

Place the baking sheets into the center of the preheated oven and bake for 12 to 15 minutes or until golden. Serve warm or at room temperature.

The chicken can be browned and stored in the refrigerator for 3 days ahead of time. Continue with the rest of the recipe as directed before serving.

# CHICKEN AND DUMPLINGS SOUP

*Makes* 6 servings

I ALMOST ALWAYS HAVE A QUART OR TWO OF THIS THICK, HOMEY CHICKEN SOUP IN THE refrigerator. Making the chicken stock and blending it with the vegetables requires very little tending, although it does require some time, so I often make the soup without the dumplings when I'm home doing other things or at night. Then I can whip up a quick batch of dumplings any time and cook them in the soup that's already been made. Just be sure to use a pot that is big enough for the dumplings to have room to swim around while they cook. They swell quite a bit.

1 recipe Chicken Stock, including chicken and vegetables (see page 26)

1¾ cups (245 g) all-purpose gluten-free flour (see page 21)

¾ teaspoon xanthan gum (omit if your blend already contains it)

¼ cup (36 g) cornstarch

4 teaspoons baking powder

½ teaspoon (3 g) kosher salt

2 eggs (100 g, weighed out of shell), at room temperature, beaten

1¼ cups (10 fluid ounces) milk, at room temperature

AFTER MAKING THE CHICKEN STOCK, REMOVE THE POT FROM THE STOVETOP. REMOVE AND discard the bay leaf. Skim any impurities off the top of the pot and discard. Remove the chicken and set it aside. Using an immersion blender, blend the vegetables used to make the stock into the liquid. Blend until no large pieces remain. Return the pot to the stovetop, and turn the heat to medium high. Cover partially and allow the liquid to come to a simmer.

In a separate medium-size bowl, blend the flour, xanthan gum, cornstarch, baking powder, and salt until well combined. Add the eggs and milk in a slow, steady stream, whisking as you go. Continue to whisk until the batter is smooth. It will be thick.

Remove the cover from the pot, and drop the dumpling batter by the heaping tablespoonful into the simmering soup, pausing in between tablespoonfuls to allow the dumplings to maintain space between one another. The dumplings swell as they cook. Cover the pot and allow the dumplings to simmer until they are cooked through, 7 to 10 minutes.

While the dumplings are cooking, remove the skin and bones from the cooked chicken from the chicken stock, and shred the meat.

Serve by ladling the soup into bowls, 2 dumplings per bowl, and topping with ½ cup shredded chicken. Serve immediately.

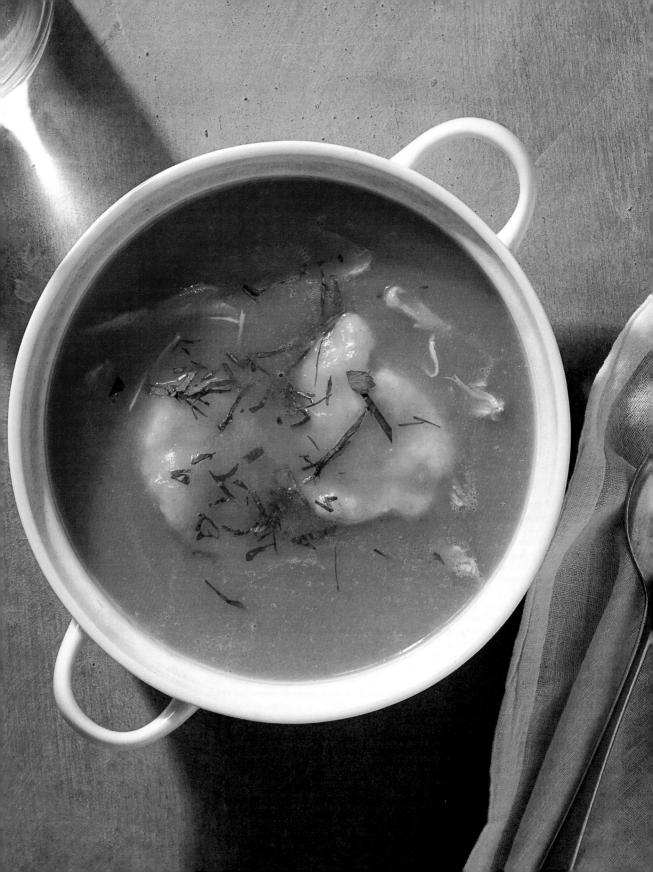

# MATZOH BALL SOUP

*Makes* 4 to 5 servings

THE NEXT TIME SOMEONE IN YOUR FAMILY IS UNDER THE WEATHER, TRY MAKING HIM or her a fresh batch of this "matzoh" ball soup. Instead of matzoh meal (the finely ground matzoh that serves as the base of many Passover dishes), it's made with quinoa flakes (which you can find at most health-food stores and many supermarkets), which means that it is not only fortified with the usual loving-kindness that comes in a warm, comforting bowl of matzoh ball soup, but it also has tons of protein. So rest up and take care. Eat, eat! You're skin and bones.

3 eggs (150 g, weighed out of shell), at room temperature, beaten

¼ cup (56 g) vegetable or other neutral oil

1 teaspoon (6 g) kosher salt

⅛ teaspoon freshly ground black pepper

1 cup quinoa flakes (plus more, if necessary, by the tablespoon)

¼ cup (36 g) all-purpose gluten-free flour (see page 21)

½ teaspoon xanthan gum (omit if your blend already contains it)

8 cups (64 fluid ounces) Chicken Stock (see page 26)

IN A LARGE BOWL, WHISK THE EGGS, OIL, SALT, AND PEPPER UNTIL WELL BEATEN. ADD THE quinoa flakes, flour, and xanthan gum, and mix to combine. If the mixture seems too squishy, add more quinoa flakes by the tablespoon until it becomes thick. Cover the bowl with plastic wrap and refrigerate for 30 minutes to an hour, until firm.

Once the mixture is firm, bring a large pot of salted water to a rolling boil. The "matzoh" balls are boiled in water, instead of in soup, because water allows them to move more freely when they cook, permitting them to cook fully, all the way through to the center of each one. Remove the batter from the refrigerator and, with wet hands, divide the mixture into 10 to 12 portions. Create round shapes of the portions by rolling them between wet palms. They will expand as they cook.

Carefully add the balls to the pot of boiling water, return to a rolling boil, cover the pot, and boil the matzoh balls for 25 to 30 minutes or until they are cooked through. You should be able to pierce each ball with a fork with little resistance. Take care not to cook so long that they begin to fall apart in the pot.

In a separate large pot, heat the chicken stock until simmering. Serve the matzoh balls in steaming bowls of chicken soup.

# TORTILLA SOUP

*Makes* 4 servings

I LOVE TAKING A BASIC DISH LIKE CHICKEN SOUP AND CLASSING IT UP A BIT. I FIND THAT it's a good way to keep the dinner doldrums at bay and also to gently diversify my children's palates. The first time I served them tortilla soup, I went light on the jalapeños, removing the seeds and the ribs and mincing the peppers very fine.

2 medium yellow onions, peeled and diced

2 tablespoons (28 g) extra-virgin olive oil

2 garlic cloves, peeled and minced

2 jalapeños, seeded and minced (remove the ribs, too, for less heat)

1 (28-ounce) can whole, peeled tomatoes, cut into chunks

3 tablespoons tomato paste

4 cups (32 fluid ounces) Chicken Stock (see page 26), including cooked chicken

½ teaspoon (3 g) kosher salt

⅛ teaspoon freshly ground black pepper

1 teaspoon ground cumin

2 to 3 tablespoons (28 to 42 g) vegetable or other neutral oil

8 corn tortillas, cut into strips ⅛ inch wide

1½ cups shredded, cooked chicken

IN A LARGE, HEAVY-BOTTOM SAUCEPAN, SAUTÉ THE ONIONS IN OLIVE OIL OVER MEDIUM-HIGH heat until translucent, about 6 minutes. Add the garlic and sauté until fragrant, about 2 minutes more.

Add the jalapeños, tomatoes, tomato paste, chicken stock, salt, pepper, and cumin. Simmer over medium heat, stirring occasionally, until thickened, about 15 minutes. Remove the skin and bones from the cooked chicken from the chicken stock recipe, and shred the meat.

Preheat the oven to 400°F. Line a rimmed baking sheet with unbleached parchment paper, and spread the strips of corn tortilla on the sheet. Toss the strips with the oil, salt, and pepper to taste. Place the baking sheet in the oven, and bake until browned, about 10 minutes, shaking the pan after 5 minutes.

Serve by ladling the soup into bowls, topping with about ½ cup of shredded, cooked chicken and a handful of tortilla strips. Serve immediately.

# POT ROAST

*Makes* 5 to 6 servings

POT ROAST IS A DELIGHTFULLY DOWN-HOME DINNER. SINCE IT'S COOKED IN SUCH DELI-ciousness for such a long time, it is foolproof to make. It can be served up simply by slicing it against the grain and drizzling it with pan juices alongside some boiled potatoes and fresh asparagus, or you can shred it with your hands and use it to make beef tacos or fajitas. You can also save whatever liquid you don't use for serving the pot roast, with all its flavors and bits and pieces of beef, and use it in place of water to make delicious brown rice. Just cook the rice according to the package directions, substituting the reserved liquid for water, one for one.

2 tablespoons (28 g) extra-virgin olive oil

4 shallots or 1 large yellow onion, peeled and diced

4 garlic cloves, crushed and peeled

1 tablespoon chipotle or red chili powder

2 tablespoons ground cumin

2 pounds beef brisket, trimmed of excess fat

2 tablespoons (36 g) kosher salt

1 tablespoon freshly ground black pepper

1 (28-ounce) can whole, peeled tomatoes, chopped

2 cups (16 fluid ounces) Chicken Stock (see page 26)

IN A VERY LARGE, HEAVY-BOTTOM POT, HEAT THE OLIVE OIL OVER MEDIUM-HIGH HEAT. ADD the shallots and garlic, and cook, stirring frequently, until the shallots are translucent and the garlic is fragrant (6 to 7 minutes). Discard the garlic. Add the chili powder and cumin, and stir to combine.

Place the brisket in the pot, and season it on all sides with the salt and pepper. Brown the brisket by rotating it in the hot pan, cooking it for about 3 to 5 minutes per side. Once the beef is browned, add the tomatoes and chicken stock, then enough water to cover the meat. Bring the liq-uid to a boil, then reduce it to a simmer, cover with the lid, and cook until the meat is very tender and begins to fall apart, about 3 ½ hours.

Once the meat is cool enough to handle, remove it from the pan and allow it to rest for 30 min-utes before slicing with a knife (against the grain) or shredding with your hands.

# CHICKEN ENCHILADAS

*Makes* 4 servings

THERE IS AN ARGUMENT TO BE MADE THAT THESE CHICKEN ENCHILADAS ARE MERELY an excuse to serve my family a ton of Easy Enchilada Sauce (see page 45), easily their favorite sauce of all. Since I make that sauce every single week without fail, this dish practically makes itself. After broiling the chicken, the dish is nearly done. Simply mix the chicken with some enchilada sauce, sour cream, beans, and cheese to make the filling. Then warm store-bought corn tortillas in a hot, dry skillet. Divide the filling among the tortillas, and pile them into a baking dish. Cover with the sauce and more cheese and bake.

1 pound boneless, skinless chicken breasts

1 teaspoon (6 g) kosher salt

⅛ teaspoon freshly ground black pepper

2 tablespoons (28 g) extra-virgin olive oil

1 recipe Easy Enchilada Sauce (see page 45)

¼ cup (64 g) sour cream

1 15-ounce can black beans, drained and rinsed

4 ounces sharp yellow Cheddar cheese, grated

6 ounces Monterey Jack cheese, grated, divided

12 corn tortillas, warmed in a hot, dry skillet until soft and pliable

PREHEAT THE OVEN TO 375°F. GREASE A 13 X 9-INCH BAKING DISH, AND SET IT ASIDE.

Place the raw chicken breasts on a large rimmed baking sheet, sprinkle evenly on both sides with the salt and pepper, and drizzle with the olive oil. Place the chicken directly under your oven's broiler for 6 minutes. Flip the breasts over and place under the broiler again for another 6 minutes or until they are cooked all the way through and reach 165°F on an instant-read thermometer. Allow the chicken to cool briefly before cutting it into a large dice.

Mix the cooked, diced chicken with ½ cup of the enchilada sauce, the sour cream, the black beans, the Cheddar cheese, and about 4 ounces of Monterey Jack cheese. Mix gently to combine. Cover the bottom of the baking dish with about ¾ cup of the enchilada sauce. Spoon some of the filling across the bottom half of a softened tortilla and roll it away from yourself until closed. Place the filled tortilla into the dish, seam-side down. Repeat with the remaining tortillas, placing them side by side in the baking dish. Pour the remaining enchilada sauce on top of all of the enchiladas, and sprinkle with the remaining 2 ounces of Monterey Jack cheese.

Place the dish in the center of the preheated oven, and bake at 375°F for about 10 minutes or until the cheese is melted and the sauce is bubbling. Serve immediately.

# ZUCCHINI-STUFFED CHICKEN PARMESAN BUNDLES

*Makes* 4 to 5 servings

A LTHOUGH I DON'T PARTICULARLY ENJOY THE PROCESS OF POUNDING CHICKEN breasts until appropriately thin, I rarely buy the thinly sliced breasts that can be used in their place. Thinly sliced breasts are only good for a few specific types of preparation, like these stuffed chicken bundles. But if you're a planner and you know what dishes you'll be making all week long, go for it. The scant 4 ounces of cream cheese make for a nice creamy richness, without any guilt. And the whole dish is still significantly easier and less messy than shallow-frying breaded chicken cutlets to make traditional chicken parmesan.

I squeeze the liquid out of grated zucchini and squash by placing it, about 1 cup at a time, in a tea towel, rolling up the towel, and twisting it to squeeze out all of the liquid. You can use whatever combination of zucchini and yellow squash you would like, or all one or the other.

½ cup (4 ounces) cream cheese, at room temperature

1 tablespoon dried oregano

1½ teaspoons dried basil

½ teaspoon (3 g) kosher salt

1 teaspoon garlic powder

8 ounces low-moisture mozzarella cheese, grated, divided

1 ounce Parmigiano-Reggiano cheese, finely grated, divided

2¼ cups zucchini and yellow squash, grated and squeezed dry of all liquid (from about 2 medium-large zucchini or squash)

1¾ pounds boneless, skinless chicken breasts, pounded to ¼ inch thickness

Egg wash (1 egg plus 1 tablespoon water, beaten)

1½ cups (180 g) gluten-free panko-style breadcrumbs (plus more if necessary)

Easy Homemade Tomato Sauce (see page 48)

12 ounces cooked gluten-free spaghetti, for serving

Chopped fresh basil, for serving

PREHEAT THE OVEN TO 375°F. LINE A LARGE RIMMED BAKING SHEET WITH UNBLEACHED parchment paper and set it aside.

In a medium-size bowl, place the cream cheese, dried oregano, and dried basil (crushed in your hands to release the oils before mixing), salt, and garlic powder, and mix to combine well. Add 6 ounces of the grated mozzarella cheese, about half of the grated Parmigiano-Reggiano cheese, and the zucchini and squash, and mix until just combined. Lay out the chicken breasts on a flat surface, divide the cream cheese and zucchini mixture among them, and spread out the mixture evenly on top of each piece of chicken. Beginning at a short end of each chicken breast, roll tightly

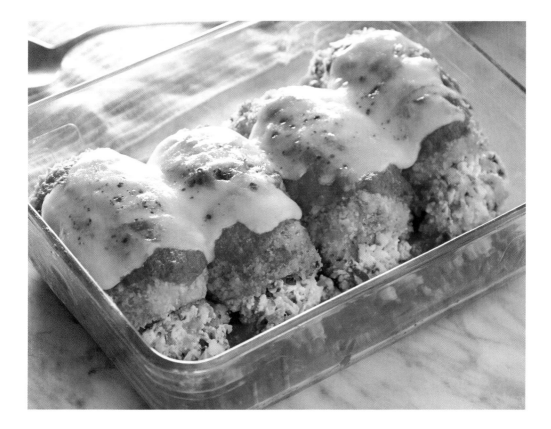

to the other end. At this point, the chicken bundles can be sealed into a freezer-safe container and frozen. Before proceeding with the recipe, defrost the chicken in the refrigerator overnight.

Before baking, set up a coating station of two shallow bowls: one with the egg wash and one with the breadcrumbs and the remaining half of the grated Parmigiano-Reggiano cheese. Next to the breadcrumbs, place the prepared baking sheet. Dredge each chicken bundle in the egg wash on all sides, allowing any excess to drip off, and then in the breadcrumb mixture on all sides, pressing the crumbs gently onto the chicken to secure them. Place the bundles, seam-side down, about an inch apart from one another on the prepared baking sheet.

Place the baking sheet in the center of the preheated oven and bake for 25 minutes. Remove from the oven, place about 2 tablespoons of tomato sauce on top of each bundle, and sprinkle with the remaining 2 ounces of grated mozzarella cheese. Return to the oven, and bake until the cheese is melted and the chicken is opaque throughout (another 5 minutes or until the chicken reaches 165°F on an instant-read thermometer). Remove from the oven, and serve over gluten-free spaghetti, sprinkled with fresh basil.

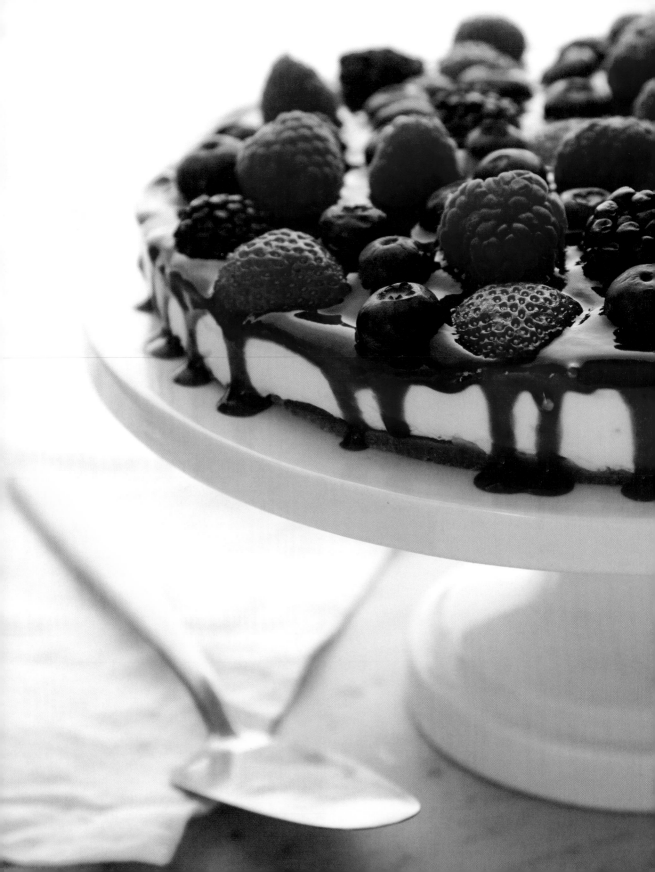

# ROOM *for* DESSERT: CAKES, COOKIES, *and* PIES

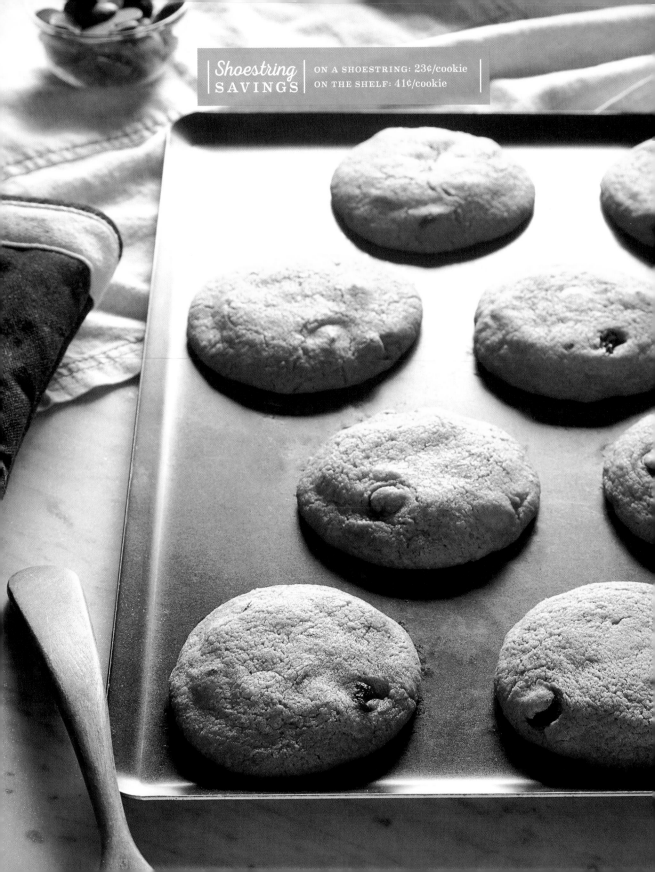

*Shoestring* SAVINGS | ON A SHOESTRING: 23¢/cookie
ON THE SHELF: 41¢/cookie

# THICK AND CHEWY
# CHOCOLATE CHIP COOKIES

*Makes* 24 cookies

I T'S REALLY IMPORTANT TO KEEP THIS BATTER COLD BEFORE YOU BAKE THESE COOKIES. That will keep them from spreading too much. You can either refrigerate the dough for an hour or so before baking or just stick the cookie sheets with the dough on them in the freezer for about 15 minutes before baking. The warmer the climate where you're baking, the longer you should refrigerate or freeze the dough before baking.

8 tablespoons (112 g) unsalted butter, at room temperature

¾ cup (150 g) granulated sugar

¾ cup (164 g) packed light-brown sugar

2 eggs (100 g, weighed out of shell), at room temperature, beaten

1 tablespoon pure vanilla extract

2¼ cups (315 g) all-purpose gluten-free flour (see page 21)

1¼ teaspoons xanthan gum (omit if your blend already contains it)

½ teaspoon (3 g) kosher salt

1 teaspoon baking soda

8 ounces semisweet chocolate chips

PREHEAT THE OVEN TO 350°F. LINE RIMMED BAKING SHEETS WITH UNBLEACHED PARCHMENT paper and set them aside.

In a large bowl, beat the butter and sugars until light and fluffy. Beat in the eggs, one at a time, and the vanilla until well blended. Add the flour, xanthan gum, salt, and baking soda to the wet ingredients, reserving a few tablespoons of dry ingredients. Mix until well combined.

In a small bowl, mix those few reserved tablespoons of dry ingredients with the chocolate chips and toss to coat. Stir the chocolate chips and the remaining dry ingredients into the cookie dough until they are evenly distributed. The dough should be very stiff and thick.

Pull off pieces of dough each about 2 tablespoons in volume. Roll each into a ball, and press into a disk about ¼ inch thick. Place about 2 inches apart on the prepared baking sheets. Place the baking sheets with the cookie dough on them into the refrigerator to chill for about 15 minutes. Once the dough has chilled, place the rimmed baking sheets in the preheated oven and bake for 7 to 10 minutes. The cookies may seem undercooked. As long as the edges are beginning to brown and the cookies are lightly browned, they're done. They will firm up. Allow to cool on the sheets for 10 minutes or until firm, then transfer to a wire rack to cool completely.

# CRISPY GINGERBREAD MEN COOKIES

*Makes* 24 5-inch-tall men

THIS IS YOUR CLASSIC GINGERSNAP COOKIE, WITH JUST ENOUGH SPICE AND THAT CRISPY cookie snap. These cookies hold their shape during baking enough to handle any gingerbread man cookie cutter or even your favorite gingerbread house template. They're also perfect for grinding into crumbs in place of Graham Crackers (see page 222) for use in a no-bake piecrust.

1½ cups (210 g) all-purpose gluten-free flour (see page 21)

¾ teaspoon xanthan gum (omit if your blend already contains it)

¼ cup (36 g) cornstarch

¾ teaspoon baking soda

1½ teaspoons ground cinnamon

1 teaspoon ground ginger

½ teaspoon (3 g) kosher salt

¼ cup (50 g) granulated sugar

⅓ cup (73 g) packed light-brown sugar

3 tablespoons (63 g) unsulfured molasses

2 tablespoons (42 g) honey

½ teaspoon pure vanilla extract

5 tablespoons (70 g) unsalted butter, at room temperature

1 egg (50 g, weighed out of shell) at room temperature, beaten

Royal Icing, for decorating (optional) (see page 262)

PREHEAT THE OVEN TO 325°F. LINE RIMMED BAKING SHEETS WITH UNBLEACHED PARCHMENT paper and set them aside.

In a large bowl, place the flour, xanthan gum, cornstarch, baking soda, cinnamon, ginger, salt, and granulated sugar, and whisk to combine well. Add the brown sugar, and whisk once more to combine, working out any lumps. Create a well in the center of the dry ingredients, and add the molasses, honey, vanilla, butter, and egg, mixing to combine after each addition. The dough will be thick and smooth and somewhat sticky to the touch.

Place the dough between two sheets of unbleached parchment paper. Roll into a rectangle about ⅜ inch thick. If you are concerned that the dough will be difficult to handle, place it in the refrigerator or freezer after you roll it out to allow it to firm up. Dip a gingerbread man cutter in all-purpose gluten-free flour or cornstarch, and use it to cut out shapes from the cookie dough. Peel back the rest of the dough from around the cutouts, and place them about 1½ inches apart on the prepared baking sheets. Gather and reroll scraps, and repeat the process until you have used all the dough.

Place the cutouts on the baking sheets in the refrigerator or freezer until firm. Place in the center of the preheated oven and bake until dry to the touch (about 15 minutes). Remove from the oven and allow to cool completely on the baking sheets. They will crisp as they cool. Decorate with the optional Royal Icing once they're completely cool.

# SOFT GINGER COOKIES

## *Makes* 24 cookies

THESE LIGHTLY SPICED COOKIES ARE ESPECIALLY PERFECT FOR THE HOLIDAYS, AS AN alternative to crispy, crunchy gingersnaps. The molasses in the cookie dough gives them depth of flavor and also helps to keep the cookies soft during baking. Pressing the pieces of raw cookie dough in sparkly coarse sugar adds a festive touch.

1½ cups (210 g) all-purpose gluten-free flour (see page 21)

¾ teaspoon xanthan gum (omit if your blend already contains it)

½ teaspoon (3 g) kosher salt

¾ teaspoon ground ginger

¼ teaspoon ground cloves

⅛ teaspoon freshly ground black pepper

½ teaspoon baking soda

½ teaspoon baking powder

¾ cup (150 g) granulated sugar

6 tablespoons (84 g) unsalted butter, at room temperature

2 tablespoons (42 g) unsulfured molasses

1 egg (50 g, weighed out of shell), at room temperature, beaten

1 teaspoon pure vanilla extract

Coarse sugar, for coating (I like Sugar in the Raw)

PREHEAT THE OVEN TO 350°F. LINE RIMMED BAKING SHEETS WITH UNBLEACHED PARCHMENT paper and set them aside.

In a large bowl, place the flour, xanthan gum, salt, ginger, cloves, pepper, baking soda, baking powder, and sugar, and whisk to combine well. Create a well in the center of the dry ingredients and add the butter, molasses, egg, and vanilla, mixing to combine after each addition. The dough will be very soft but should hold together well and be smooth. Transfer the dough to a large piece of unbleached parchment paper and shape into a cylinder about 1½ inches in diameter. Roll the cylinder tightly in the parchment, rocking it back and forth to create a proper cylinder shape, then twist the ends to seal. Place the shaped dough on a flat surface, and place in the freezer to chill for about 10 minutes or until firm enough to slice.

Place the dough on a cutting surface, rock it back and forth to round the bottom edge again, and unwrap the dough. Using a sharp knife and a smooth motion, slice the dough by cross-section into 24 equal pieces, each about ¼ inch thick. Press each of the pieces of dough into the coarse sugar firmly enough for the sugar to adhere to the cookie dough on all sides of each piece. Place about 2½ inches apart from one another on the prepared baking sheets.

Place the baking sheets, one at a time, in the center of the preheated oven and bake until lightly golden brown all over and set in the center, about 10 minutes. Remove from the oven and allow to cool on the baking sheet for about 5 minutes or until firm before transferring to a wire rack to cool completely.

# SOFT FROSTED
# SUGAR COOKIES

### *Makes* 30 cookies

THESE SOFT AND BUTTERY SUGAR COOKIES HOLD THEIR SHAPE IN THE OVEN AND DON'T even need to be chilled before baking. The edges stay clean whether you're baking them as rounds or a festive holiday shape. These are the cookies that you can use for every single holiday and occasion throughout the year. The frosting stays firm at room temperature because of the addition of meringue powder. LorAnn Oils brand meringue powder is readily available and reliably gluten-free. A small jar lasts a long time.

COOKIES

2 cups (280 g) all-purpose gluten-free flour (see page 21)

1 teaspoon xanthan gum (omit if your blend already contains it)

¾ teaspoon baking powder

½ teaspoon (3 g) kosher salt

½ cup (100 g) granulated sugar

3 tablespoons (22 g) confectioners' sugar

8 tablespoons (112 g) unsalted butter, at room temperature

1 egg (50 g, weighed out of shell), at room temperature, beaten

½ teaspoon pure vanilla extract

FROSTING

10 tablespoons (140 g) unsalted butter, at room temperature

¼ cup milk (2 fluid ounces), at room temperature

1 tablespoon pure vanilla extract

⅛ teaspoon (almost 1 g) kosher salt

2 teaspoons meringue powder

4 cups (460 g) confectioners' sugar

PREHEAT THE OVEN TO 350°F. LINE RIMMED BAKING SHEETS WITH UNBLEACHED PARCHMENT paper and set them aside.

In a large bowl, place the flour, xanthan gum, baking powder, salt, granulated sugar, and confectioners' sugar, and whisk to combine well. Add the butter, egg, and vanilla, and mix to combine. The dough will be thick and relatively stiff, and you may need to squeeze it together with your hands to bring all of it together.

Roll the dough between two sheets of unbleached parchment paper into a round a bit less than ⅓ inch thick. Using a 2 ½-inch round cookie cutter, cut out rounds of dough and place them about 1 inch apart on the prepared baking sheets.

Place the baking sheet in the center of the preheated oven and bake until just set, about 6 minutes. The edges of some of the cookies may brown slightly. Remove the cookies from the oven before they brown and allow them to cool until set. Transfer to a wire rack to cool completely.

While the cookies are cooling, make the frosting. In the bowl of your stand mixer fitted with the paddle attachment or a large bowl with a handheld mixer, place the butter, milk, and vanilla, and mix on medium speed until combined. Turn the speed up to high, and mix until creamy. Add the salt, meringue powder, and about 3 ½ cups of confectioners' sugar. Mix slowly until the sugar is incorporated. Turn the mixer up to high, and beat until it becomes uniformly thick. Add the rest of the confectioners' sugar if necessary to thicken the frosting.

Once the cookies are completely cool, pipe or spoon a generous amount of frosting onto the top of each, and spread into an even layer with a wide knife or offset spatula. Allow to set at room temperature until the frosting hardens a bit. Store any leftovers in an airtight container at room temperature.

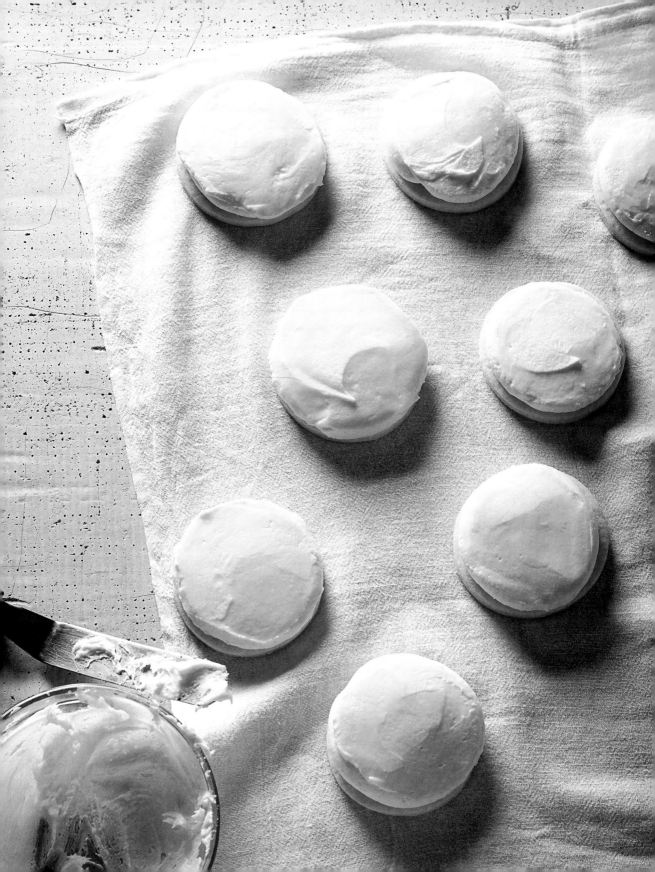

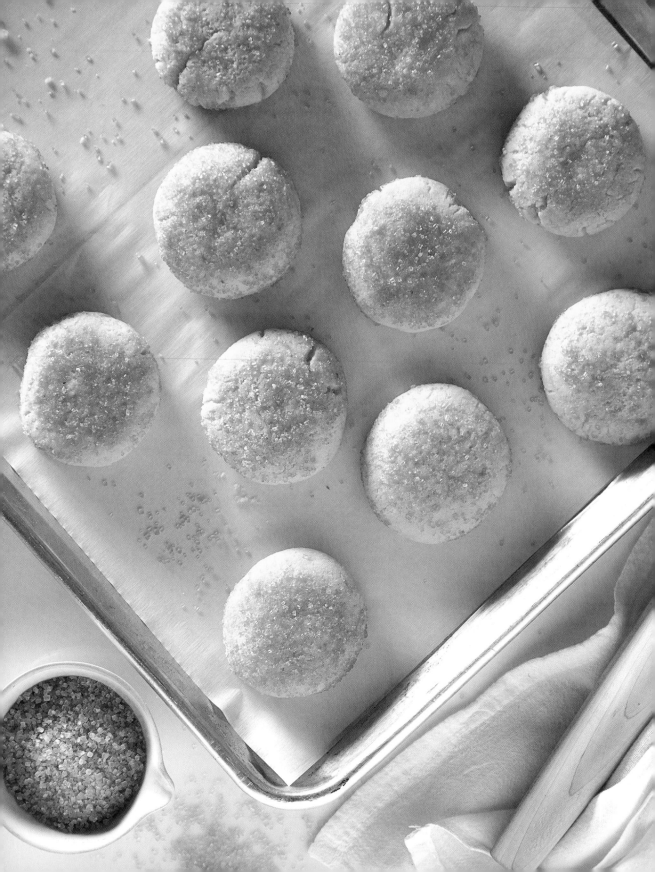

# DROP SUGAR COOKIES

*Makes* 18 cookies

W HEN YOU DON'T FEEL LIKE ROLLING OUT COOKIE DOUGH AND CUTTING OUT shapes, quick and easy drop sugar cookies are what you want. You can dress them up a bit by rolling them in a festive-colored coarse sugar instead of Sugar in the Raw.

1 ¾ cups (245 g) all-purpose gluten-free flour (see page 21)

¾ teaspoon xanthan gum (omit if your blend already contains it)

1 teaspoon baking powder

½ teaspoon (3 g) kosher salt

½ cup (58 g) confectioners' sugar

½ cup (100 g) granulated sugar

5 tablespoons (70 g) unsalted butter, at room temperature

5 tablespoons (60 g) vegetable shortening, melted and cooled

1 egg (50 g, weighed out of shell), at room temperature, beaten

2 teaspoons pure vanilla extract

Coarse sugar, for coating (I like Sugar in the Raw)

PREHEAT THE OVEN TO 350°F. LINE A RIMMED BAKING SHEET WITH UNBLEACHED PARCHMENT paper and set it aside.

In a large bowl, place the flour, xanthan gum, baking powder, salt, confectioners' sugar, and granulated sugar, and whisk to combine well. Add the butter, shortening, egg, and vanilla, mixing well to combine after each addition. The dough should come together and will be soft. Roll the dough into balls about 1 inch in diameter, and press into disks about ¼ inch thick. Press each disk carefully but firmly into coarse sugar until the sugar adheres to the dough all around. Place the disks of dough on the prepared baking sheet, about 1 inch apart from one another.

Place in the center of the preheated oven and bake for 10 minutes or until lightly golden brown on the edges and set in the center. Remove from the oven and allow to cool on the baking sheet for 5 minutes before transferring to a wire rack to cool completely.

*Shoestring* SAVINGS | ON A SHOESTRING: 20¢/cookie
ON THE SHELF: 39¢/cookie

# CRISPY CHOCOLATE
# WAFER COOKIES

*Makes* 48 cookies

THESE ARE THE CRISPY-CRUNCHY, DEEP CHOCOLATE WAFER COOKIES THAT USUALLY come in a sleeve. They're perfect for layering with fresh whipped cream for an icebox cake or sandwiching together with a chocolate sandwich cookie filling (see page 220). They're also very useful for crushing into crumbs and using for a no-bake piecrust.

1¾ cups (245 g) all-purpose gluten-free flour

¾ teaspoon xanthan gum (omit if your blend already contains it)

½ cup (40 g) unsweetened natural cocoa powder

⅛ teaspoon baking soda

¾ cup (150 g) granulated sugar

½ teaspoon (3 g) kosher salt

8 tablespoons (112 g) unsalted butter, at room temperature

1 egg (50 g, weighed out of shell), at room temperature, beaten

1½ teaspoons pure vanilla extract

PREHEAT THE OVEN TO 325°F. LINE RIMMED BAKING SHEETS WITH UNBLEACHED PARCHMENT paper and set them aside.

In a large bowl, place the flour, xanthan gum, cocoa powder, baking soda, sugar, and salt, and whisk to combine well. Add the butter, egg, and vanilla, and mix until the dough comes together. It will be thick and smooth. Divide the dough into two equal parts, and roll each out between two sheets of unbleached parchment paper until the dough is ⅛ inch thick (the thickness of a nickel), no thinner.

Pull back the top sheet of parchment paper on one piece of dough. Flour a round 2¼-inch cookie cutter, and use it to cut out rounds. Transfer the rounds to the prepared baking sheets, and place them about 1 inch apart (they will not spread much during baking). Gather and reroll the scraps, and cut more rounds. Repeat with the second piece of dough.

Place the baking sheets, one at a time, in the center of the preheated oven and bake until the cookies spring back when pressed lightly in the center (about 8 minutes).

Remove the baking sheet from the oven, and allow cookies to cool on the baking sheet until firm. Transfer to a wire rack to cool completely. To maintain texture, store in a sealed glass container at room temperature.

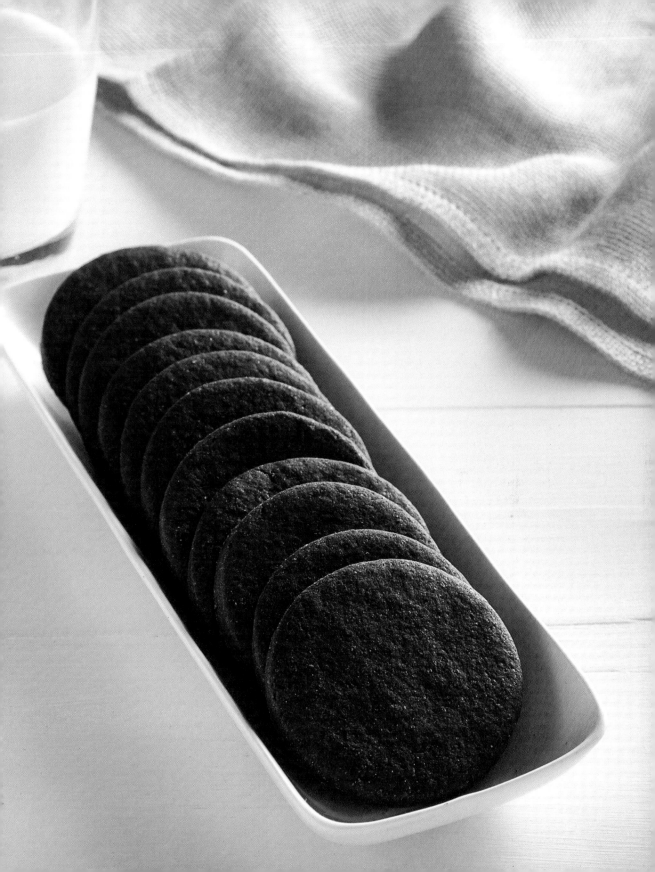

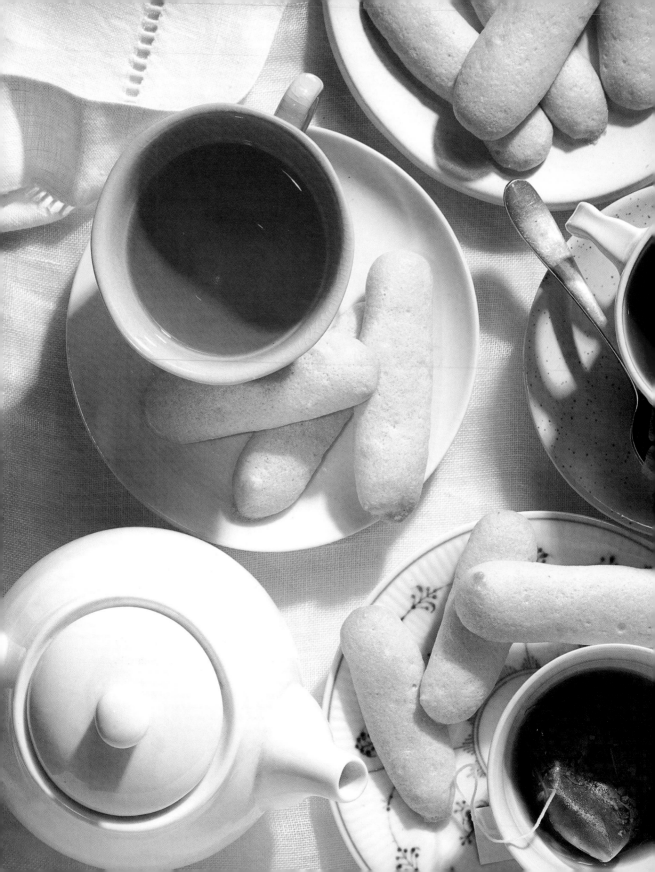

# LADYFINGERS

*Makes* about 12 ladyfingers

Ladyfingers are not just for ladies. And they're not actual fingers. They're just vaguely reminiscent of fingers in their shape. They are delicate and lightly sweet, with a thin, crispy outside and a light and cakey inside, like angel food cake. These elegant little cookies are easy on the wallet, too, because they don't use much flour.

4 eggs (200 g), separated into yolks and whites

⅛ teaspoon cream of tartar

½ cup (58 g) confectioners' sugar

¾ cup (105 g) all-purpose gluten-free flour (see page 21)

½ teaspoon xanthan gum (omit if your blend already contains it)

½ teaspoon (3 g) kosher salt

1½ teaspoons pure vanilla extract

PREHEAT THE OVEN TO 325°F. LINE TWO BAKING SHEETS WITH UNBLEACHED PARCHMENT paper and set them aside.

In the bowl of your stand mixer fitted with the whisk attachment or a large bowl with a handheld mixer, beat the egg whites and the cream of tartar until stiff, but not dry, peaks form. Gently scrape the whites out of the bowl of the mixer into another medium bowl and set them aside.

In the bowl of your stand mixer (or the same large bowl with a handheld mixer), beat the egg yolks and the sugar for 8 to 10 minutes on at least medium speed, until pale yellow, thick, and nearly tripled in volume.

Into the yolk mixture, gently fold the flour, xanthan gum, salt, and vanilla, and then the egg white mixture, until smooth.

Fill a pastry bag fitted with a ¾-inch plain tip (or a zip-top plastic bag with a hole cut in the corner) with the dough. Pipe fingers about 4 inches long, 2 inches apart, on the prepared baking sheets. Place the baking sheets in the preheated oven and bake for about 12 to 15 minutes, until pale golden on the outside, rotating the sheets halfway through baking.

Remove from the oven and allow the ladyfingers to cool until firm on the baking sheets. To maintain texture, store in a sealed glass container at room temperature. These will not maintain their texture when frozen.

*Shoestring* SAVINGS | ON A SHOESTRING: 14¢/cookie
ON THE SHELF: 33¢/cookie

# CHOCOLATE CHIP BISCOTTI

*Makes* 20 to 24 cookies

ISCOTTI IS THE SORT OF CRISPY, CRUNCHY COOKIE THAT JUST SEEMS SO QUINTESSEN-tially gluten containing to me. So I think it's important to serve a nice batch of these twice-baked, no-butter cookies to any friends or family members who are still skeptical that foods can be both gluten-free and delightfully tasty. Nothing is entirely out of reach. Who needs gluten?

1½ cups (210 g) all-purpose gluten-free flour (see page 21)

¾ teaspoon xanthan gum (omit if your blend already contains it)

1 teaspoon baking powder

½ teaspoon (3 g) kosher salt

½ cup (100 g) granulated sugar

5 ounces semisweet chocolate chips

2 eggs (100 g, weighed out of shell), at room temperature, beaten

1 tablespoon pure vanilla extract

PREHEAT THE OVEN TO 350°F. LINE A RIMMED BAKING SHEET WITH UNBLEACHED PARCHMENT paper and set it aside.

In a large bowl, place the flour, xanthan gum, baking powder, salt, and sugar, and whisk to combine well. Add the chocolate chips, and mix to combine. Add the eggs and vanilla extract, and mix to combine well. The dough will be thick and sticky. If necessary to bring it together, knead the dough with wet hands until smooth.

Place the dough in the center of the prepared baking sheet, and shape with wet hands into a loaf that is approximately 7 inches long, 3 inches wide, and 1 inch thick. Place in the center of the preheated oven and bake until lightly golden brown and firm to the touch, about 20 minutes. Remove from the oven and allow the loaf to cool for at least 10 minutes or until only slightly warm to the touch. Lower the oven temperature to 300°F.

Slice the loaf in cross-section on the bias into 10 to 12 pieces, each about ¼ inch thick. Place the pieces back on the prepared baking sheet, flat and spaced about 1 inch apart. Return the baking sheet to the oven and bake for 10 minutes. Flip each of the cookies over on the baking sheet; return to the oven and finish baking until the underside of the cookies is lightly golden brown (about another 10 minutes—less if you want less crunchy cookies). Remove from the oven and allow to cool to room temperature before serving. The cookies will crisp as they cool.

Store biscotti at room temperature in a sealed glass container at room temperature for about 3 days.

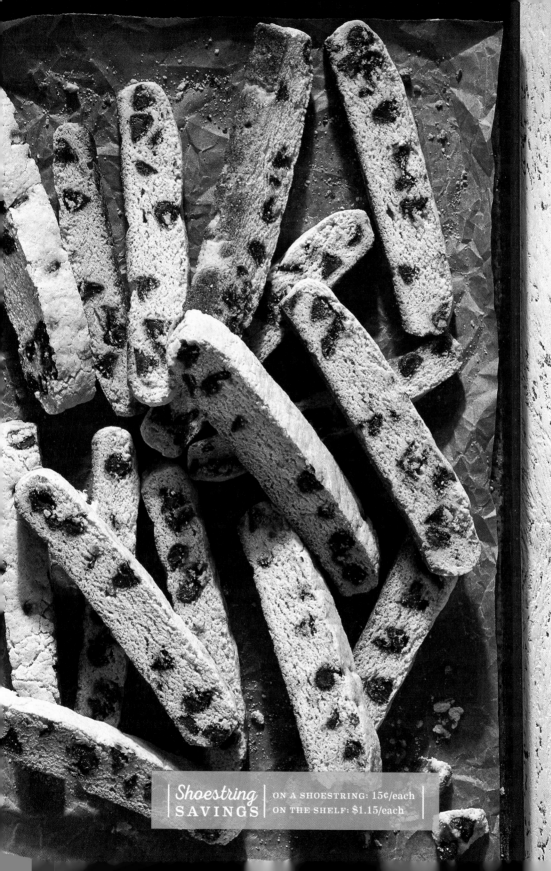

*Shoestring* SAVINGS | ON A SHOESTRING: 15¢/each
ON THE SHELF: $1.15/each

# BLACK AND WHITE COOKIES

*Makes* about 16 cookies

T HESE COOKIES ARE A NEW YORK FAVORITE, AND WHENEVER I SEE ANYONE TRY TO PASS off a cookie as a black and white when it is frosted, rather than iced, I take personal offense. The icing should be thick enough that it dries opaque but thin enough that it dribbles slowly off a spoon. You'll need to make the cookies well in advance of icing them because they must be completely cool or the icing will stay wet and weepy, and you won't get a smooth finish because the cookies will crumble when you try to ice them. The cookies themselves are worth eating on their own, but nothing compares to a beautiful, iced black and white.

### COOKIES

5 tablespoons (70 g) unsalted butter, at room temperature

½ cup (100 g) granulated sugar

1 egg (50 g, weighed out of shell), at room temperature, beaten

½ teaspoon pure vanilla extract

⅓ cup (85 g) sour cream, at room temperature

1¼ cups (175 g) all-purpose gluten-free flour (see page 21)

½ teaspoon xanthan gum (omit if your blend already contains it)

½ teaspoon baking soda

½ teaspoon (3 g) kosher salt

### ICING

1½ cups (173 g) confectioners' sugar (plus more by the tablespoon)

1 tablespoon light corn syrup

1 teaspoon freshly squeezed lemon juice

¼ teaspoon vanilla extract

¼ cup (20 g) unsweetened cocoa powder

PREHEAT THE OVEN TO 350°F. LINE RIMMED BAKING SHEETS WITH UNBLEACHED PARCHMENT paper and set them aside.

In a large bowl, place the butter and sugar, and beat until light and fluffy. Add the egg, then the vanilla and sour cream, beating well in between each addition. Add the flour, xanthan gum, baking soda, and salt, and mix to combine. Chill the batter before baking it to keep the cookies from spreading too much. Spoon the chilled batter onto the lined baking sheets by the heaping tablespoonful, about 2 inches apart.

Place in the center of the preheated oven, and bake until the cookie tops are puffed and pale golden, about 15 minutes. Allow to cool completely on the baking sheet.

To make the icing, in a medium-size bowl, place the confectioners' sugar, corn syrup, lemon juice, vanilla, and about 1 tablespoon of water. Mix until completely smooth. Transfer half the icing into another medium-size bowl, add the cocoa, and stir very well. Add water by the tablespoonful to thin (or more confectioners' sugar to thicken, also by the tablespoonful) both the black and the white icing separately, stirring very well after each addition. The consistency should be such that it dribbles from a spoon gracefully, like molasses.

To ice the cookies, turn them flat side up, and spread the white icing over half and the black over the other half. The icing should be thick enough that it doesn't melt into the cookie when you spread it. If it disappears, add some more confectioners' sugar and stir to thicken. Allow to set before serving.

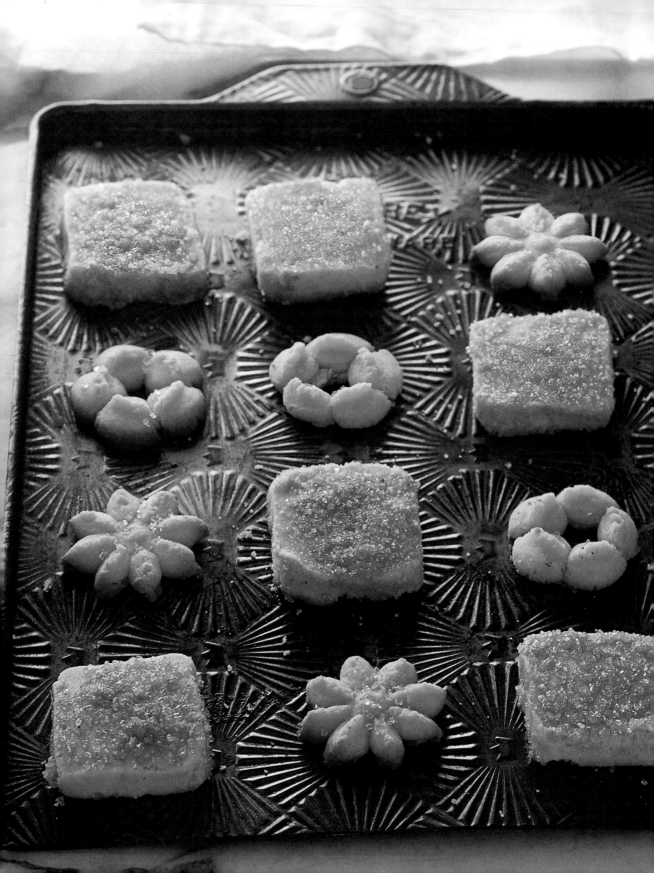

# BUTTER COOKIES

*Makes* about 40 cookies, depending upon size

**B**UTTER COOKIES ARE LOVELY, DELICATE LITTLE CREATIONS, PERFECT FOR HIGH TEA, and they make an amazing crust for cheesecake (see page 230). Years ago, I thought it would be brilliant to cut this dough with cookie cutters in the shape of letters in order to spell out a congratulatory message to one of my children. It wasn't. So if you ever find yourself in need of cookies as a means of communication, use the Soft Frosted Sugar Cookies (page 203) instead. They're much more robust. You could probably even write a short story out of sugar cookies. Butter cookies are more refined, so be kind to them. This is the recipe that you use to make spritz butter cookies if you enjoy using a cookie press, or simple icebox cookies that are shaped into a rectangle and chilled and sliced before baking.

| | |
|---|---|
| 1½ cups (210 g) all-purpose gluten-free flour (see page 21) | 8 tablespoons (112 g) unsalted butter, at room temperature |
| ¾ teaspoon xanthan gum (omit if your blend already contains it) | 3 egg yolks (75 g, weighed out of shell), at room temperature |
| ½ cup plus 2 tablespoons (72 g) confectioners' sugar | 1 teaspoon pure vanilla extract |
| ½ teaspoon (3 g) kosher salt | 1 extra egg white plus coarse sugar (I like Sugar in the Raw) for decorating (optional) |

PREHEAT THE OVEN TO 350°F.

In the bowl of a food processor fitted with the metal blade, place the flour, xanthan gum, sugar, and salt, and pulse to combine well. One at a time, add the butter, egg yolks, and vanilla, pulsing to combine after each ingredient. Pulse again until the dough comes together in a ball. The dough should be smooth and a bit wet, but you should be able to handle it lightly.

For spritz cookies, do not chill the dough. It must be room temperature to adhere to the baking sheet. Fill your cookie press according to the manufacturer's directions. You will want to form half the dough into a cylinder a bit smaller than the size of the chamber, then slide the dough in. Place the disk you like on the end of the chamber, and screw the end on securely.

On a bare, ungreased baking sheet that is *not* nonstick, dispense the cookie dough, spacing it evenly. I have the most luck getting the cookie shape to stick to the sheet when I place the press firmly onto the surface, press the lever on the press until I feel some resistance, hold steady, and then release quickly.

For icebox cookies, wrap the dough in plastic wrap and shape it into a cylinder about 1½ inches in diameter. Square each of the sides with a straight edge to form a rectangle, and place the log in the refrigerator or freezer until firm (about 15 minutes in the refrigerator or 5 minutes in the freezer). Unwrap the chilled log, and slice into cross-section pieces about ¼ inch wide. Place the cookies evenly spaced on a lined baking sheet.

With a pastry brush, brush the tops of all of the cookies on the baking sheet with the egg white and sprinkle with coarse sugar, for optional decorating.

Place the baking sheet in the center of the preheated oven and bake, rotating once, until just beginning to turn lightly brown around the edges, about 8 minutes. Allow to cool completely on the pan before moving the cookies, or they will break.

| *Shoestring* SAVINGS | ON A SHOESTRING: 8¢/cookie |
| | ON THE SHELF: 44¢/cookie |

# COOKIE BREAKUP

*Makes* about 24 "cookies,"
depending upon size

THESE COOKIES TASTE EVEN BETTER FROZEN. EATEN RIGHT FROM THE BAG. BEFORE the freezer door closes. (Hypothetically.) And they can be made super quick, so they're a great thing to throw together if you are looking for a last-minute host(ess) gift to bring to someone's house. Just don't forget to suggest to your host(ess) that he or she siphon off a few and stick 'em in the freezer for late-night hankerings.

12 tablespoons (168 g) unsalted butter, at room temperature

1 cup (200 g) granulated sugar

½ teaspoon (3 g) kosher salt

1 teaspoon pure vanilla extract

2 cups (280 g) all-purpose gluten-free flour (see page 21)

1 teaspoon xanthan gum (omit if your blend already contains it)

8 ounces semisweet chocolate chips

PREHEAT THE OVEN TO 350°F. LINE A 13 × 9-INCH RIMMED BAKING SHEET WITH UNBLEACHED parchment paper and set it aside.

In a large bowl, place the butter and sugar, and beat until light and fluffy. Add the salt and vanilla, and beat to combine. Add the flour and xanthan gum to the batter, reserving a few tablespoons of the flour. Mix to combine. The dough should stick together well when pressed in your palm. Toss the chocolate chips in the reserved flour until the chips are coated. Add the chocolate chips and reserved flour to the batter, and stir until the chips are evenly distributed throughout the dough.

Press the dough into the prepared baking sheet in an even layer, ensuring it all sticks together, and then place it in the center of the preheated oven. Bake for 12 to 15 minutes or until just beginning to brown around the edges. Allow the panel of cookies to cool completely on the sheet before breaking it into irregular shapes.

# CHOCOLATE SANDWICH COOKIES

*Makes* about 30 cookies

T HESE OTHERWISE SIMPLE COOKIES HAVE A BIG WOW FACTOR. THEY'RE ADDICTIVE BUT not in the same way as a certain famous chocolate sandwich cookie. Eating an entire sleeve of those cookies makes me feel vaguely ashamed. But baking and then eating a bunch of these, the homemade gluten-free version, makes me feel clever, ingenious even.

4 tablespoons (56 g) unsalted butter, at room temperature

4 tablespoons (48 g) nonhydrogenated vegetable shortening

1¼ teaspoons pure vanilla extract

1 to 1½ cups (115 to 173 g) confectioners' sugar

1 recipe Crispy Chocolate Wafer Cookies (see page 208)

IN A LARGE BOWL, PLACE THE BUTTER, SHORTENING, AND VANILLA, AND BEAT UNTIL WELL blended. Add 1 cup of confectioners' sugar, and stir until the sugar is incorporated completely into the butter mixture. The filling should be thick and stiff. Add more confectioners' sugar, one tablespoon at a time, to reach the desired consistency.

Place one-half of the chocolate wafer cookies upside down on a level surface. Divide the filling among the cookies, and flatten with wet hands or a spoon. Place the other half of the cookies right-side up on top of the filling, and press down gently to create sandwich cookies.

# CHEWY SUGAR COOKIES

*Makes* about 20 cookies

SIMILAR TO THE DROP SUGAR COOKIES ON PAGE 207, THERE IS NO ROLLING INVOLVED IN making these cookies. These spread significantly in the oven, though. The result is a lovely thin and chewy sugar cookie with a delicate, buttery taste.

1½ cups (210 g) all-purpose gluten-free flour (see page 21)

¾ teaspoon xanthan gum (omit if your blend already contains it)

2 tablespoons (18 g) cornstarch

½ teaspoon baking soda

¼ teaspoon baking powder

½ teaspoon (3 g) kosher salt

1 cup (200 g) granulated sugar

6 tablespoons (84 g) unsalted butter, at room temperature

2 tablespoons (24 g) nonhydrogenated vegetable shortening, melted and cooled

1 egg (50 g, weighed out of shell), at room temperature, beaten

1 teaspoon pure vanilla extract

PREHEAT THE OVEN TO 300°F (NOT A TYPO!). LINE RIMMED BAKING SHEETS WITH UNBLEACHED parchment paper and set them aside.

In a large bowl, place the flour blend, xanthan gum, cornstarch, baking soda, baking powder, salt, and sugar, and whisk to combine well. Create a well in the center of the dry ingredients, and add the butter, shortening, egg, and vanilla, mixing to combine after each addition. The dough will be thick and smooth but easy to shape and not greasy (unless you didn't allow the shortening to cool after melting it!).

Divide the dough into 20 pieces, and roll each into a ball (about 1 inch in diameter). Press each ball of dough into a disk about ⅜ inch thick, and place fully 2 inches apart from one another on the prepared baking sheets. The cookies will spread quite a lot during baking.

Place the baking sheets in the freezer to chill until firm (about 5 minutes). Remove from the freezer, and place in the center of the preheated oven and bake until set in the center and just beginning to brown around the edges (about 12 minutes). Remove from the oven, and allow to cool on the baking sheet for at least 10 minutes, or until stable, before transferring to a wire rack to cool completely.

# GRAHAM CRACKERS

*Makes* about 20 crackers

Without graham crackers, there are no s'mores, and there is no graham cracker crust. Without graham cracker crust, you can't make a proper Banana Cream Pie (see page 247). These crackers are lightly sweet, keep beautifully in a sealed glass container, and can be made into any shape you like, although I keep it old school: perforated rectangles.

2 cups (280 g) all-purpose gluten-free flour (see page 21), plus more for sprinkling

1 teaspoon xanthan gum (omit if your blend already contains it)

¼ teaspoon baking soda

¼ teaspoon baking powder

⅛ teaspoon (almost 1 g) kosher salt

1 teaspoon ground cinnamon

¼ cup (50 g) granulated sugar

⅓ cup (72 g) packed light-brown sugar

6 tablespoons (72 g) nonhydrogenated vegetable shortening, melted and cooled

2 tablespoons (42 g) honey

2 tablespoons (42 g) unsulfured molasses

½ teaspoon pure vanilla extract

1 egg (50 g, weighed out of shell), at room temperature, beaten

2 to 4 tablespoons (1 to 2 fluid ounces) milk, at room temperature

Preheat the oven to 325°F. Line rimmed baking sheets with unbleached parchment paper and set them aside.

In a large bowl, place the flour, xanthan gum, baking soda, baking powder, salt, cinnamon, and granulated sugar, and whisk to combine well. Add the brown sugar, and whisk again, working out any lumps. Create a well in the center of the dry ingredients, and add the shortening, honey, molasses, vanilla, egg, and 2 tablespoons of the milk, mixing to combine after each addition. Knead the dough with your hands, adding more milk 1 teaspoonful at a time as necessary to bring the dough together.

Transfer the dough to a lightly floured piece of unbleached parchment paper and, sprinkling lightly with flour as necessary to prevent sticking, roll out the dough until it is about ¼ inch thick. Using a pastry wheel, pizza cutter, or sharp knife, trim any rough edges, and then cut the dough into 4 × 2-inch shapes. Place the shapes about 1 inch apart from one another on the prepared baking sheets. Gather and reroll the scraps to cut out more until you've used up the dough. Using the tines of a fork, pierce each piece of dough about 4 times. For an authentic touch, score each rectangle of dough by slicing about halfway through the dough across, widthwise.

Place the baking sheets, one at a time, in the center of the preheated oven, and bake until the crackers are golden brown all over and firm to the touch, about 15 minutes. Remove from the oven and allow to cool completely on the baking sheets. They will crisp as they cool.

To maintain texture, store in a sealed glass container at room temperature.

*Shoestring*
SAVINGS

ON A SHOESTRING: 18¢/ounce
ON THE SHELF: 69¢/ounce

# LEMON CUPCAKES

*Makes* 12 cupcakes

THESE CUPCAKES ARE A REFRESHING ALTERNATIVE TO YELLOW CUPCAKES, WITH OR without the Citrus Glaze (see page 260). Since they are very moist, they freeze quite nicely, so there are always a few of these in our deep freezer. When I get last-minute notice of an upcoming birthday party in my son's school, I just grab one of these out of the freezer, stick it in a container, and stash it in his backpack without even defrosting it. It's ready to go when the party gets started.

8 tablespoons (112 g) unsalted butter, at room temperature

1 cup (200 g) granulated sugar

2 eggs (100 g, weighed out of shell), at room temperature, beaten

1½ teaspoons pure vanilla extract

Zest and juice of 1 lemon (reserve 1 to 2 tablespoons for glaze)

1½ cups (210 g) all-purpose gluten-free flour (see page 21)

¾ teaspoon xanthan gum (omit if your blend already contains it)

2 teaspoons baking powder

½ teaspoon (3 g) kosher salt

½ cup (113 g) sour cream, at room temperature

Citrus Glaze (see page 260) (optional)

PREHEAT THE OVEN TO 350°F. GREASE OR LINE A STANDARD 12-CUP MUFFIN TIN AND SET IT ASIDE.

In a large bowl, place the butter and sugar, and beat until light and fluffy. Add the eggs, vanilla, lemon zest, and juice (reserving the final 1 to 2 tablespoons of juice for the glaze), mixing to combine after each addition. Add the flour, xanthan gum, baking powder, and salt, and mix to combine. Add the sour cream to the batter and mix until combined.

Divide the batter evenly among the muffin cups and bake in the center of the preheated oven for about 25 minutes, until a toothpick inserted into the center of a cupcake comes out clean. Cool for 5 minutes in the tin and then transfer to a wire rack to cool completely. Glaze once cooled.

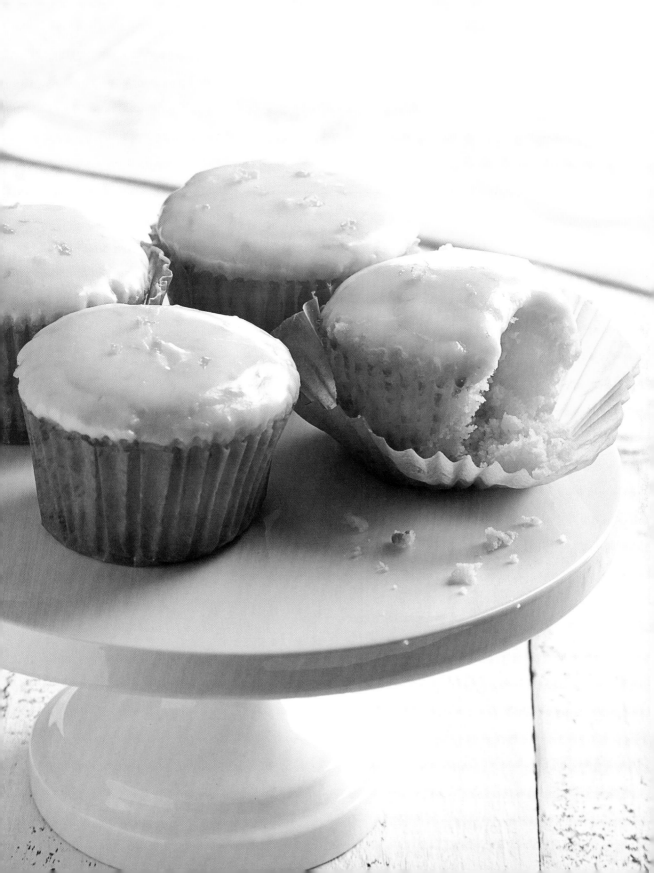

# CHOCOLATE CHIP
# BLONDIE CUPCAKES

*Makes* 12 cupcakes

THE BROWN SUGAR IN THESE BLONDE-BROWNIE CUPCAKES MAKES THEM A DENSER AND more decadent alternative to traditional vanilla and chocolate cupcakes.

8 tablespoons (112 g) unsalted butter, at room temperature

1½ cups (327 g) packed light-brown sugar

2 eggs (100 g, weighed out of shell), at room temperature, beaten

2 teaspoons pure vanilla extract

2 cups (280 g) all-purpose gluten-free flour (see page 21)

1 teaspoon xanthan gum (omit if your blend already contains it)

½ teaspoon baking soda

½ teaspoon (3 g) kosher salt

1 cup (6 ounces) semisweet chocolate chips

PREHEAT THE OVEN TO 350°F. GREASE OR LINE A STANDARD 12-CUP MUFFIN PAN AND SET IT ASIDE.

In a large bowl, place the butter and sugar together, and mix until light and fluffy. Add the eggs and the vanilla, and mix to combine.

To the large bowl of wet ingredients, add the flour, xanthan gum, baking soda, and salt, reserving a few tablespoons of the dry ingredients in a small bowl, and mix to combine. Add the chocolate chips to the reserved dry ingredients, and toss to coat them, then add them to the batter, and stir to distribute the chips evenly throughout.

Divide the batter evenly among the prepared wells of the muffin tin. The batter should be thick and stiff.

Place the muffin pan in the preheated oven and bake for 20 to 22 minutes, until a toothpick inserted in the center of a cupcake comes out clean. Remove from the oven and allow to cool in the baking pan for 10 minutes before transferring to a wire rack to cool completely.

# CHOCOLATE CHIP BROWNIES

*Makes* 16 brownies

W E COULDN'T VERY WELL HAVE A COOKBOOK OF BASICS WITHOUT HAVING A RECIPE for basic, chewy brownies. These are your classic brownies, dense, rich, and chewy as the day is long.

8 tablespoons (112 g) unsalted butter, at room temperature

2 cups (12 ounces) semisweet chocolate chips, divided

1¼ cups (250 g) granulated sugar

3 eggs (150 g, weighed out of shell), at room temperature, beaten

1 cup (140 g) all-purpose gluten-free flour (see page 21)

½ teaspoon xanthan gum (omit if your blend already contains it)

¼ cup (20 g) unsweetened natural cocoa powder

¼ teaspoon baking powder

⅛ teaspoon baking soda

½ teaspoon (3 g) kosher salt

PREHEAT THE OVEN TO 350°F. LINE AN 8-INCH SQUARE BAKING PAN WITH TWO CRISSCROSSED strips of unbleached parchment paper long enough to overhang all the sides of the pan. Set the pan aside.

In a medium-size microwave-safe bowl, place the butter and 8 ounces of chocolate chips. Microwave for 1½ to 2 minutes, 30 seconds at a time, stirring well after each 30-second interval, until the chocolate is melted and smooth. Allow the chocolate mixture to cool slightly, for about 2 minutes.

Once the chocolate mixture has cooled, add the sugar and the eggs, one at a time, mixing to combine after each addition. Add the flour, xanthan gum, cocoa powder, baking powder, baking soda, and salt, reserving a few tablespoons of flour and mixing to combine after each addition. Toss the remaining 4 ounces of chocolate chips with the reserved flour to coat the chocolate chips. Add the chocolate chips and remaining flour to the batter, stirring until the chips are evenly distributed throughout the batter. Scrape the batter into the prepared pan, and smooth the top with a wet spatula.

Place the pan in the preheated oven and bake for 25 to 30 minutes, until a toothpick inserted into the center comes out mostly clean, with a few moist crumbs attached. Cool the brownies in the pan for at least 30 minutes. Lift the brownies out of the pan with the overhung parchment paper, invert onto a cutting board, peel off the parchment paper, and slice into squares with a moistened serrated knife.

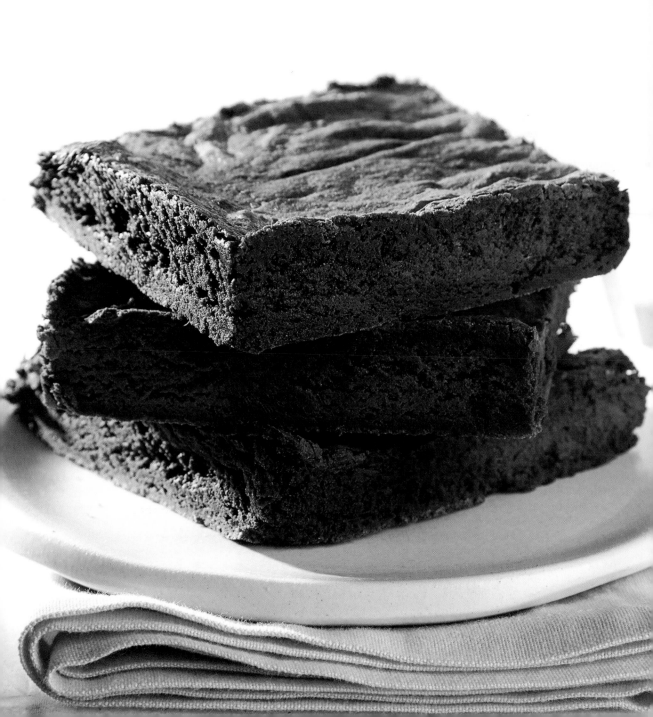

# FLOURLESS BROWNIES

*Makes* 9 to 12 brownies, depending upon size

I F RICH AND FUDGY BROWNIES ARE WHAT YOU CRAVE, THESE FLOURLESS BROWNIES ARE for you. There's nothing cake-like about them. For a paleo version of these amazing brownies, replace the butter with an equal amount of virgin coconut oil and the granulated sugar with an equal amount of coconut palm sugar.

10 ounces dark chocolate, chopped

4 tablespoons (56 g) unsalted butter, chopped

¾ cup (150 g) granulated sugar

3 eggs (150 g, weighed out of shell), at room temperature

2 teaspoons pure vanilla extract

¼ cup (20 g) unsweetened cocoa powder (Dutch-processed is preferred but not essential)

½ teaspoon (3 g) kosher salt

PREHEAT THE OVEN TO 350°F. GREASE AND LINE AN 8-INCH SQUARE BAKING PAN WITH UNbleached parchment paper that overhangs the sides of the pan, and set it aside.

In a double boiler or a medium-size microwave-safe bowl, melt the chocolate and butter or coconut oil until melted and smooth. To melt the chocolate in the microwave, heat in 30-second increments at 70 percent power, stirring in between intervals, taking care not to burn the chocolate. To the melted chocolate and butter mixture, add the sugar, mix to combine well, and then set the bowl aside. In a separate, large bowl, place the eggs and vanilla, and beat with a hand mixer on medium-high speed until frothy (about 1 minute). Add the cocoa powder and salt to the eggs, and beat on low speed until the cocoa powder is absorbed (about 1 minute). Add the chocolate and butter mixture to the large bowl, and beat on medium-high speed until the mixture is smooth and glossy (2 to 3 minutes).

Pour the mixture into the prepared baking pan, spread it into an even layer, and tap the pan on a flat surface to break any large air bubbles. Place the pan in the center of the preheated oven, and bake until set in the center (22 to 25 minutes). Do not overbake. Remove the pan from the oven, place it on a wire rack, and allow to cool completely.

Lift the brownies from the pan by the overhung parchment paper, and place on a cutting board. Slice the brownies into 9 or 12 equal parts with a sharp, wet knife, lift and serve.

# NO-BAKE CHEESECAKE

*Makes* one 9-inch cheesecake

A NO-BAKE CHEESECAKE IS LOVELY FOR THE WARM WEATHER, WHEN YOU DON'T FEEL like turning on the oven. This cheesecake is made with low-fat Greek yogurt in place of some of the cream cheese and is lighter in sugar than you might expect. Be sure not to skip the gelatin, or the cheesecake won't set up. If you don't have a springform pan, you can use a 9-inch round or square pan lined with unbleached parchment paper, which overhangs the sides of the pan.

### CRUST

1½ cups (225 g) gluten-free cookie crumbs (like crushed Graham Crackers [see page 222])

5 tablespoons (70 g) virgin coconut oil or unsalted butter, melted and cooled

### FILLING

1 cup (227 g) low-fat (or nonfat) plain Greek yogurt, at room temperature

¼ cup (2 fluid ounces) cool water

1 teaspoon (3 g) unflavored powdered gelatin

¼ teaspoon cream of tartar (or 1 teaspoon light corn syrup)

2 (8-ounce) packages cream cheese, at room temperature

⅛ teaspoon kosher salt

¾ cup (86 g) confectioners' sugar

1½ teaspoons pure vanilla extract

Seeds from 1 vanilla bean (optional)

GREASE A 9-INCH SPRINGFORM PAN AND SET IT ASIDE. IN A MEDIUM-SIZE BOWL, PLACE THE cookie crumbs and melted coconut oil or butter, and mix until all of the crumbs are moistened. Place the cookie crumb mixture in the prepared pan, and press firmly into an even layer on the bottom of the pan and very slightly up the sides. Place the pan in the freezer for about 15 minutes or until the crust is firm.

Place the Greek yogurt in a strainer over an empty bowl, and allow the yogurt to drain for at least a few minutes. In a small saucepan or heat-safe bowl, place the cool water and sprinkle the gelatin on top in an even layer. Allow the mixture to sit for a few minutes until the gelatin swells. Heat the mixture over low heat or in the microwave for about 20 seconds or until the gelatin is dissolved and the mixture has liquefied. Add the cream of tartar or corn syrup, and mix to combine. Remove the gelatin mixture from the heat, and allow to cool until no longer hot to the touch. In the bowl of a stand mixer fitted with the paddle attachment or a large bowl with a hand

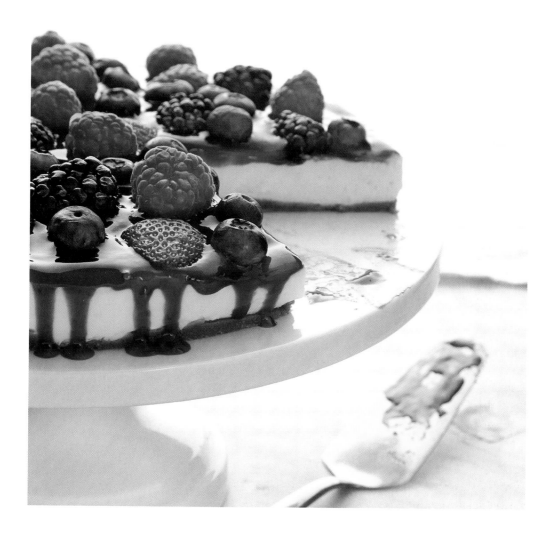

mixer, place the cream cheese, drained Greek yogurt, salt, confectioners' sugar, vanilla extract, and optional vanilla seeds, beating to combine well after each addition. While beating slowly, add the dissolved gelatin mixture in a slow drizzle, and continue to beat until the mixture begins to thicken (about 5 minutes).

Pour the filling mixture into the chilled crust and spread into an even layer. Place the cheesecake in the refrigerator until set (about 3 hours). To serve, unmold the cheesecake or lift the cake out of the 9-inch round or square pan by the overhung parchment paper. Cut into wedges or squares and serve chilled.

# PERFECT YELLOW CAKE

*Makes* two 8-inch round cakes

THIS IS THE VANILLA, OR YELLOW, CAKE TO END ALL YELLOW CAKES. THE CRUMB IS impossibly tender, with just enough vanilla flavor to satisfy. It's not heavy or dense, but each moist bite simply melts in your mouth. I enjoy chocolate as much as the next girl, but I'm a vanilla cake lover at heart. This is the cake I choose for every occasion, every single time. You simply must sift the flour, starch, and leaveners, the butter and sugar must be beaten well first, and this cake cannot be made in one bowl. Every step counts. As written, the recipe makes two 8-inch round cakes, with 4 egg whites and 1 whole egg. To halve the recipe, use 3 egg whites (75 g) in place of the 4 egg whites and 1 whole egg. Half of the recipe can also be used to make yellow cupcakes. Divide the batter evenly among the 12 wells of a standard muffin tin and bake as directed but for about 20 minutes.

2 cups (280 g) all-purpose gluten-free flour (see page 21)

1 teaspoon xanthan gum (omit if your blend already contains it)

¼ cup plus 2 tablespoons (54 g) cornstarch

½ teaspoon baking soda

2 teaspoons baking powder

½ teaspoon (3 g) kosher salt

10 tablespoons (140 g) unsalted butter, at room temperature

1½ cups (300 g) granulated sugar

2 teaspoons pure vanilla extract

4 egg whites (100 g) plus 1 egg (50 g, weighed out of shell), at room temperature

1⅓ cups (10⅔ fluid ounces) buttermilk, at room temperature

PREHEAT THE OVEN TO 350°F. GREASE TWO 8-INCH ROUND CAKE PANS AND LINE THE BOTTOM of each with a round of unbleached parchment paper (trace the perimeter of the cake pan on the parchment, then cut out the circle). Set the pans aside.

Into a medium-size bowl, sift the flour, xanthan gum, cornstarch, baking soda, and baking powder. Add the salt, and whisk to combine well. Set the dry ingredients aside. In the bowl of a stand mixer fitted with the paddle attachment or a large bowl with a handheld mixer, beat the butter, sugar, and vanilla on medium-high speed for at least 3 minutes, stopping at least once to scrape the entire mixture off the sides and bottom of the bowl, or until very light and fluffy. Combine the egg whites, egg, and buttermilk in a small bowl, and whisk to combine well. To the large bowl with the butter and sugar mixture, add the dry ingredients in 4 equal portions, alternating with the buttermilk and egg mixture in 3 parts, beginning and ending with the dry ingredients and mixing to combine in between additions. The batter will sometimes look a bit curdled. Once

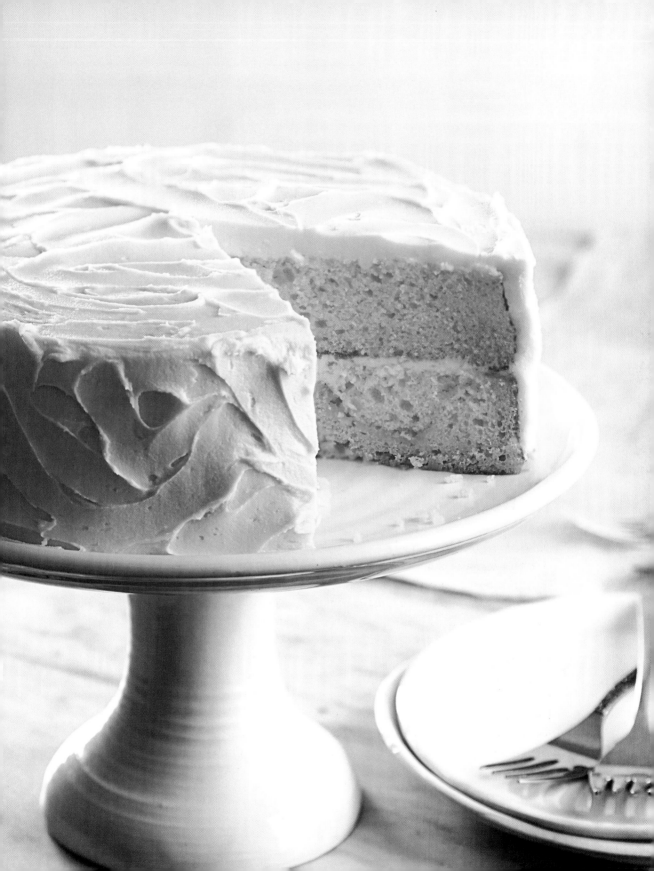

all of the ingredients have been added, beat for another minute on medium speed to ensure that everything is combined, and then turn over the batter a few times by hand. It should be very thick but pourable and relatively smooth.

Divide the batter evenly between the two prepared baking pans, and smooth each into an even layer with an offset spatula. Place the baking pans in the center of the preheated oven, and bake for 20 minutes. Rotate the pans, and continue to bake until the cakes are lightly golden brown all over, have begun to pull away from the sides of the pan, and do not jiggle in the center at all (about another 10 minutes). I find that these tests for doneness are more useful than the toothpick test.

Remove the cakes from the oven, and allow to cool in the pans for 15 minutes before turning out onto a wire rack (and removing the parchment paper liners) to cool completely before frosting and serving.

*Shoestring*
SAVINGS | ON A SHOESTRING: 24¢/each when made as cupcakes
ON THE SHELF: $1.45/each cupcake

# DEVIL'S FOOD CAKE

*Makes* two 8-inch round cakes or 24 cupcakes

I F A DEVIL'S FOOD SNACK CAKE IS WHAT YOU CRAVE, A SNACK CAKE YOU SHOULD HAVE. Simply bake this cake in a square pan. While the cake is cooling, whip up a batch of the filling from Chocolate Sandwich Cookies (see page 220). Once the cake has cooled, turn it over and slice it carefully in the middle with a large serrated knife, creating two equal rectangles. Spread the sandwich cookie filling evenly over the bottom of one of the rectangles, top with the other rectangle, and slice into individual snack cakes. If you get caught in the act, just say, "The Devil made me do it."

2 cups (280 g) all-purpose gluten-free flour (see page 21)

1 teaspoon xanthan gum (omit if your blend already contains it)

¾ cup (60 g) unsweetened natural cocoa powder

1¼ teaspoons baking soda

½ teaspoon (3 g) kosher salt

1½ cups (327 g) packed light-brown sugar

1⅓ cups (10⅔ fluid ounces) warm water

8 tablespoons (112 g) unsalted butter, at room temperature

½ cup (113 g) sour cream, at room temperature

2 eggs (100 g, weighed out of shell), at room temperature, beaten

1 teaspoon pure vanilla extract

PREHEAT THE OVEN TO 325°F. GREASE TWO 8-INCH ROUND CAKE PANS OR LINE TWO STANDARD 12-cup muffin tins with liners. Set the pans aside.

In a large bowl, place the flour, xanthan gum, cocoa powder, baking soda, and salt, and whisk to combine well. Add the brown sugar, and whisk again to combine, working out any lumps in the sugar. Create a well in the center of the dry ingredients, and add the water, butter, sour cream, eggs, and vanilla, mixing to combine after each addition. The batter will be soft and relatively thick. Divide the batter evenly between the 2 prepared baking pans, or fill the wells of each muffin cup about ¾ of the way with batter. Smooth the tops of the batter.

Place the baking pans at the same time, or the muffin tins one at a time, in the center of the preheated oven. If making cakes, bake for 15 minutes, rotate the pans, and continue to bake until the tops spring back when pressed lightly and a toothpick inserted in the center comes out with a few moist crumbs attached (about another 10 minutes). If making cupcakes, bake until the tops of the cupcakes spring back when pressed lightly (about 22 minutes). Remove from the oven, and allow to cool for 10 minutes in the tin before transferring to a wire rack to cool completely.

# POUND CAKE

## *Makes* 1 cake

THIS POUND CAKE MAY REMIND YOU OF A CERTAIN BRAND-NAME POUND CAKE THAT can be found in the freezer aisle. Packaged in a foil pan with a cardboard cover, it was always in my sweet-toothed grandmother's freezer (I realize that the part about my grandmother is not a helpful part of the hint for most of you). But this one's gluten-free, and you can make it at home for a fraction of the cost. It can be made up to 3 days ahead of time, wrapped tightly, and stored at room temperature until ready to serve. It also freezes quite well and can even be drizzled with Citrus Glaze (see page 260).

16 tablespoons (224 g) unsalted butter, at room temperature

1 cup (200 g) granulated sugar

4 extra-large or 5 large eggs (250 g, weighed out of shell), at room temperature, beaten

2 teaspoons pure vanilla extract or 1½ teaspoons vanilla extract plus ½ teaspoon almond extract

1¼ cups (175 g) all-purpose gluten-free flour (see page 21)

½ teaspoon xanthan gum (omit if your blend already contains it)

¼ cup plus 1 tablespoon (45 g) cornstarch

1 teaspoon (6 g) kosher salt

PREHEAT THE OVEN TO 325°F. GREASE WELL A STANDARD LOAF PAN (ABOUT 9 × 5 INCHES OR A bit smaller) and set it aside.

In the bowl of a stand mixer fitted with the paddle attachment or a large bowl with a handheld mixer, cream the butter on medium-high speed until it is light and fluffy. Add the sugar, and then the eggs (slowly, while the mixer is on low speed) and vanilla, beating after each addition until well combined. Turn the mixer speed up to medium high, and beat until smooth.

In a small bowl, place the flour blend, xanthan gum, cornstarch, and salt, and whisk to combine well. Add the flour mixture, about ¼ cup at a time, to the mixer bowl with the wet ingredients, and mix until just combined. The batter will be thick but soft and smooth. Scrape the mixture into the prepared loaf pan, and smooth the top with a wet spatula. Carefully bang the bottom of the pan a few times on the counter to release any air bubbles.

Place the loaf pan in the center of the preheated oven and bake, rotating once during baking, until lightly golden brown all over and a toothpick inserted in the center comes out clean (about 50 minutes). Remove from the oven and place the cake, still in the pan, on a wire rack to cool for at least 30 minutes before removing from the pan and allowing to cool completely.

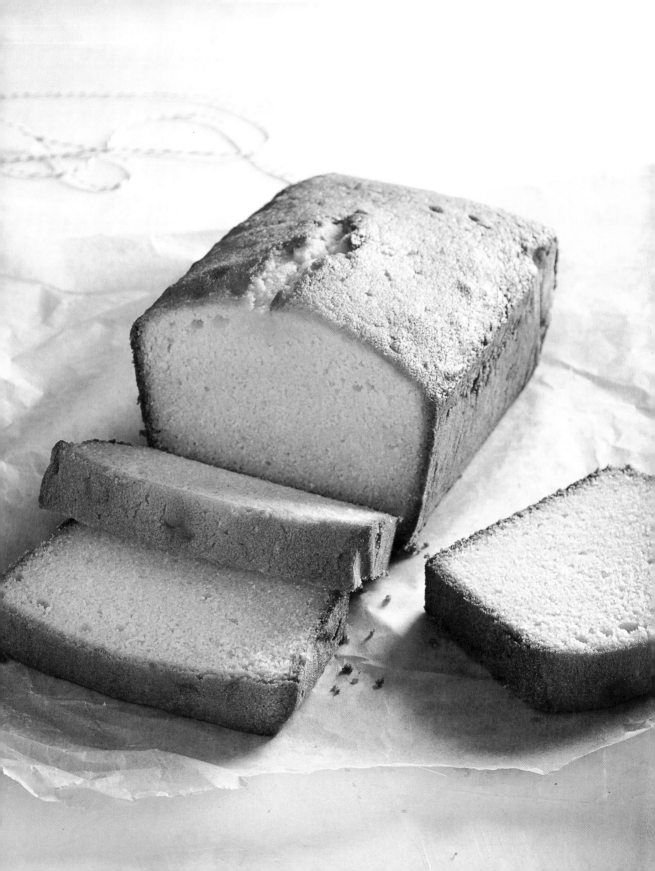

# PERFECT CHOCOLATE BIRTHDAY CAKE

*Makes* one 9-inch round cake
or 18 cupcakes

THIS CAKE IS A REAL CROWD-PLEASER. EVERYONE SEEMS TO BE ABLE TO AGREE UPON IT. Typically, to make a rich chocolate cake, you need to replace some of the butter with melted chocolate. In this cake, though, there's nearly a full cup of cocoa powder. Combined with a neutral oil, the cocoa powder makes for a very deep chocolate cake.

1 cup plus 2 tablespoons (157 g) all-purpose gluten-free flour (see page 21)

½ teaspoon xanthan gum (omit if your blend already contains it)

⅞ cup (70 g) unsweetened natural cocoa powder

1 teaspoon baking powder

½ teaspoon baking soda

½ teaspoon (3 g) kosher salt

1⅛ cups (225 g) granulated sugar

6 tablespoons (84 g) vegetable or other neutral oil

3 eggs (150 g, weighed out of shell), at room temperature, beaten

¾ cup (6 fluid ounces) lukewarm water

PREHEAT THE OVEN TO 350°F. GREASE OR LINE A STANDARD 12-CUP MUFFIN TIN OR 9-INCH cake pan and set it aside.

In a large bowl, place the flour, xanthan gum, cocoa powder, baking powder, baking soda, salt, and sugar, and whisk to combine well. Create a well in the center, and add the oil, eggs, and water, mixing to combine well after each addition.

Fill the prepared wells of the cupcake tin ⅔ of the way full or transfer the cake batter to the prepared round pan and smooth the top with a wet spatula. Place in the center of the preheated oven, and bake until a toothpick inserted in the center comes out mostly clean or with a few moist crumbs attached (about 19 minutes for cupcakes; about 28 minutes for the cake).

Remove from the oven and allow to sit in the pan for at least 10 minutes before transferring to a wire rack to cool completely. For the cupcakes, repeat with the remaining batter.

# APPLE CAKE

*Makes* 12 to 15 squares of apple cake

A NICE WARM, BUTTERY APPLE CAKE LIKE THIS ONE IS AN ESSENTIAL PART OF YOUR repertoire. It may be less iconic than an apple pie and not quite as effortless to throw together as apple crisp—however, you'll find that people tend to fall naturally into three separate and distinct categories: you have your crisp people, your pie people, and your cake people. I want to make sure that like a Boy (or Girl) Scout, you're prepared for any eventuality.

CAKE

12 tablespoons (168 g) unsalted butter, at room temperature

1½ cups (300 g) granulated sugar

2 eggs (100 g, weighed out of shell), at room temperature, beaten

1 tablespoon pure vanilla extract

2 cups (280 g) all-purpose gluten-free flour (see page 21)

1 teaspoon xanthan gum (omit if your blend already contains it)

1 teaspoon baking soda

½ teaspoon (3 g) kosher salt

2 teaspoons ground cinnamon

⅓ cup (76 g) sour cream, at room temperature

FILLING

3 to 4 firm apples, peeled, cored, and sliced thin (Granny Smith work well here)

¼ cup plus 1 tablespoon (63 g) granulated sugar

¼ cup plus 1 tablespoon (68 g) packed light-brown sugar

2 teaspoons ground cinnamon

¼ teaspoon kosher salt

1 teaspoon (3 g) cornstarch

PREHEAT THE OVEN TO 325°F. GREASE OR LINE A 13 × 9-INCH BAKING DISH WITH UNBLEACHED parchment paper and set it aside.

In a large bowl, cream the butter and sugar until light and fluffy. Add the eggs and vanilla, and beat to combine. Add the flour, xanthan gum, baking soda, salt, and cinnamon, beating well after each addition. Add the sour cream and blend. Set aside to prepare the filling.

In a separate, medium-size bowl, place the apples, sugars, cinnamon, salt, and cornstarch, and stir to combine well.

Layer one-half of the cake batter evenly in the prepared baking dish, then layer in the filling mixture and top evenly with the remaining cake batter, smoothing the top with wet hands.

Place the baking dish in the center of the preheated oven and bake for 45 minutes to 1 hour or until a toothpick inserted in the center comes out clean.

Cool completely in the dish. Remove the cake from the pan, and slice it into squares with a serrated knife.

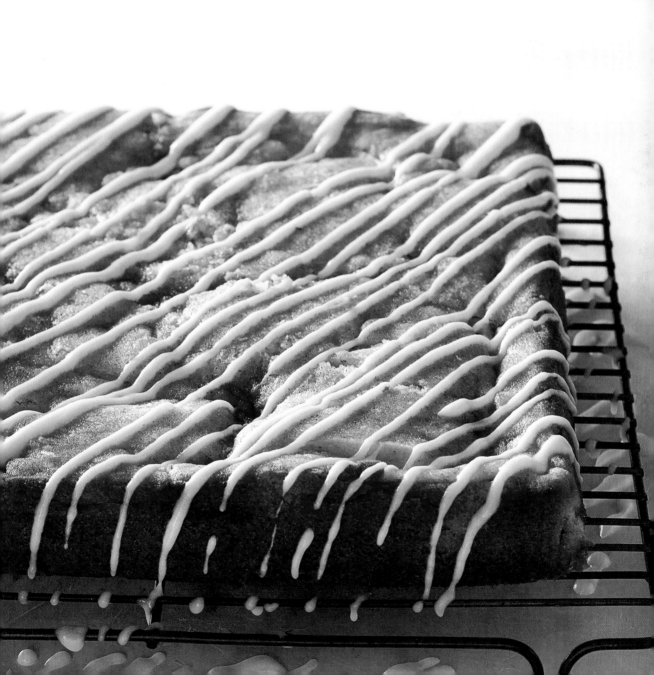

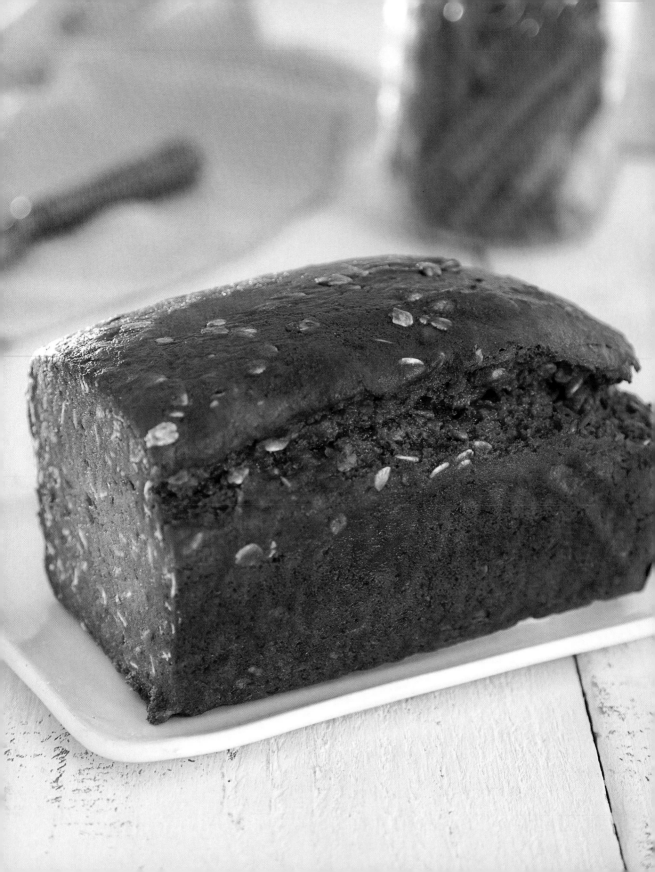

# PUMPKIN BREAD

*Makes* 1 loaf

THIS IS A VERY MOIST AND FLAVORFUL QUICK BREAD THAT IS GREAT FOR THANKSGIVING but works all year-round. All you have to do is stock up on packed pumpkin in November, and you'll be ready at a moment's notice, any time of year.

2 cups (280 g) all-purpose gluten-free flour (see page 21)

1 teaspoon xanthan gum (omit if your blend already contains it)

¾ cup (150 g) granulated sugar

¾ cup (75 g) certified gluten-free old-fashioned rolled oats

1½ teaspoons baking soda

1 teaspoon ground cinnamon

1½ cups (366 g) canned packed pumpkin

¾ cup (252 g) pure maple syrup

2 tablespoons (28 g) neutral oil

2 egg whites (50 g, weighed out of shell), at room temperature

7 pitted prunes

2 to 3 tablespoons (1 to 1½ fluid ounces) lukewarm water

½ cup raisins (soaked in warm water for 15 minutes, then drained)

PREHEAT OVEN TO 350°F. GREASE OR LINE A 9 × 5-INCH LOAF PAN AND SET IT ASIDE.

In a large bowl, place the flour, xanthan gum, sugar, oats, baking soda, and cinnamon. Whisk to combine. Add the pumpkin, maple syrup, oil, and egg whites, mixing to combine well after each addition. In a blender or food processor, place the prunes and lukewarm water, and purée until smooth. Add to the batter, and mix to combine. Add the raisins, and mix until evenly distributed throughout the batter.

Scrape the batter into the prepared loaf pan, and smooth the top with a wet spatula. Place in the preheated oven, and bake for about 1 hour, until a toothpick inserted into the center of the loaf pan comes out mostly clean or with a few moist crumbs attached. Remove from the oven, and allow to cool in the pan for 15 minutes before transferring to a wire rack to cool completely. Slice and serve.

# PUMPKIN CHOCOLATE CHIP SQUARES

*Makes* about 9 squares

I CAME CLOSE TO SETTING THIS RECIPE ASIDE, THINKING THAT WE HAD ENOUGH PUMPKIN-laden, Thanksgiving-themed recipes for one cookbook. And then one day my son asked my husband what his favorite dessert was. Imagine my surprise when he answered, "Pumpkin Chocolate Chip Squares." So that settled it. These squares are worth squirreling away a few cans of packed pumpkin in the fall for other times of year. Pumpkin pairs remarkably well with chocolate. Try to resist the (understandable) temptation, though, to add more pumpkin than the recipe calls for. It really throws off the moisture balance in the squares and makes them gooey, but in a bad way.

8 tablespoons (112 g) unsalted butter, at room temperature

⅝ cup (125 g) granulated sugar

1 egg (50 g, weighed out of shell), at room temperature, beaten

2 teaspoons pure vanilla extract

½ cup (122 g) canned solid packed pumpkin

1 cup (140 g) all-purpose gluten-free flour (see page 21)

½ teaspoon xanthan gum (omit if your blend already contains it)

2 teaspoons pumpkin pie spice

½ teaspoon baking soda

½ teaspoon (3 g) kosher salt

1 cup (6 ounces) semisweet chocolate chips

PREHEAT THE OVEN TO 350°F. LINE A 9-INCH SQUARE BAKING PAN WITH UNBLEACHED PARCH-ment paper, allowing the lining to overhang the edges. Set aside.

In a large bowl, beat the butter and sugar until light and fluffy. Add the egg, then the vanilla and pumpkin, and beat to combine. Add the flour, xanthan gum, pumpkin pie spice, baking soda, and salt, beating after each addition until combined, reserving a couple tablespoons of the flour in a small bowl. Add the chocolate chips to the small bowl of reserved flour, and toss to coat. Then add the flour-coated chips to the batter, and stir until the chips are evenly distributed throughout.

Scrape the batter into the prepared baking pan, smoothing the top. Place the pan in the pre-heated oven, and bake until a toothpick inserted into the center of the pan comes out mostly clean or with a few moist crumbs attached (about 25 minutes).

Allow to cool completely in the pan. Once cool, lift out the squares by the overhung parchment paper. Peel back the parchment paper, and slice into squares with a serrated knife.

# PUMPKIN PIE WITH
# GINGER COOKIE CRUST

*Makes* 8 servings

SAY FAREWELL TO THE OBLIGATORY THANKSGIVING PUMPKIN PIE THAT BARELY GETS touched except by your one great aunt who demands that you make it, fusses over it noisily, and then eats only a sliver. The smooth, sweet filling of this pie, made from the flesh of a freshly baked sugar pumpkin (a small and round pumpkin, with sweet, dark orange flesh) blended with rich evaporated milk, is balanced to perfection by the aromatic crust that is crisp but not brittle. The depth of flavor that comes from homemade roasted pumpkin is really worth the trouble. If you'd prefer to use canned packed pumpkin purée instead, you'll need 13 ounces for the filling.

CRUST

½ cup (70 g) all-purpose gluten-free flour (see page 21)

¼ teaspoon xanthan gum (omit if your blend already contains it)

⅓ cup (67 g) granulated sugar

2 cups finely ground Crispy Gingerbread Men Cookies (see page 202)

8 tablespoons (112 g) unsalted butter, melted and cooled

¼ cup pumpkin purée (from baked sugar pumpkin in filling, ingredients)

FILLING

1 sugar pumpkin (cut, seeded, and baked for 40 minutes at 350°F, the flesh puréed until smooth)

2 eggs (100 g, weighed out of shell)

1 cup (218 g) packed light-brown sugar

1 tablespoon (9 g) all-purpose gluten-free flour (see page 21)

½ teaspoon (3 g) kosher salt

2½ teaspoons pumpkin pie spice

1 can (12 fluid ounces) evaporated milk

TO MAKE THE CRUST, GREASE A 9-INCH PIE PLATE WITH UNSALTED BUTTER AND SET IT ASIDE.

In a medium-size bowl, stir together the flour, xanthan gum, granulated sugar, cookie crumbs, butter, and pumpkin purée, and blend well. Press the mixture into the bottom and sides of the pie plate. Cover with plastic wrap and chill for at least 1 hour. Before the crust is ready to be baked, preheat the oven to 325°F. Remove the plastic wrap from the pie shell, cover the crust with foil to prevent burning, place it in the preheated oven, and bake for 10 minutes.

To make the filling, preheat the oven to 450°F. In a large bowl, combine the remaining pumpkin purée, the eggs, brown sugar, flour, salt, pumpkin pie spice, and evaporated milk, blending well after each addition. Pour the filling into the cooled, baked shell. Place the pie in the preheated oven, and bake for 10 minutes, and then turn down the oven temperature to 350°F and bake for another 45 to 60 minutes, or until a toothpick inserted into the center of the pie comes out clean.

Cool the pie to room temperature, cover with plastic wrap, and refrigerate overnight. Serve chilled.

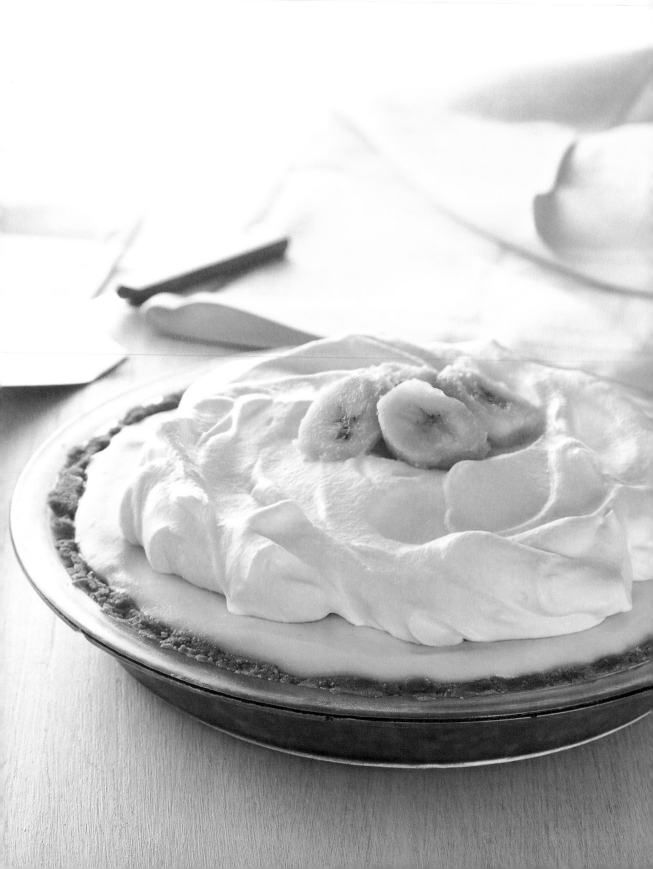

# BANANA CREAM PIE
# WITH GRAHAM CRACKER CRUST

*Makes* 8 servings

THIS BANANA CREAM PIE IS EASY AS ONE, TWO, THREE, BUT IT DOES TAKE AT LEAST that many steps. It's a special pie for a special occasion because it requires deliberate advance planning. Even the graham cracker crust is extraordinary: the addition of a mashed banana makes the crust slightly moist and chewy.

CRUST

2 cups finely ground Graham Crackers (see page 222)

⅓ cup (67 g) granulated sugar

1 banana (100 g), peeled and mashed

6 tablespoons (84 g) unsalted butter, melted and cooled

FILLING

½ cup (100 g) granulated sugar

⅓ cup (48 g) cornstarch

½ teaspoon (3 g) kosher salt

½ cup (4 fluid ounces) heavy whipping cream, at room temperature

2½ cups (20 fluid ounces) milk, at room temperature

3 egg yolks (75 g, weighed out of shell), at room temperature

1½ teaspoons pure vanilla extract

FOR LAYERING

4 ripe (but not overripe) bananas, sliced in ¼-inch disks

TO MAKE THE CRUST, PREHEAT THE OVEN TO 350°F. GREASE WELL A 10-INCH PIE PLATE AND set it aside.

In a medium-size bowl, stir together the graham cracker crumbs, sugar, banana, and butter, and mix well. Press the cracker mixture into the bottom and sides of the pie plate. Cover with plastic wrap and chill for at least 10 minutes or until firm. Once chilled, remove the plastic wrap from the pie shell, place it in the preheated oven, and bake for 10 to 12 minutes or until pale golden. Cool the crust completely.

To make the pie filling, in a medium saucepan, whisk together the sugar, cornstarch, and salt. Without turning on the heat, gradually add the cream and milk in a steady stream, and then the egg yolks one at a time, whisking constantly. Place the saucepan on the stovetop, and turn on the heat to medium, still whisking constantly, and cook for about 7 minutes or until the mixture begins to thicken.

Remove the saucepan from the heat and add the vanilla extract, whisking to combine. Pour the custard into a large, flat bowl, place plastic wrap directly on the surface of the custard, and allow it to sit at room temperature until it has cooled, about 1 hour.

Once the custard has cooled completely, remove the plastic wrap and stir if necessary to smooth the consistency. Pour 1 cup of the custard on top of the graham cracker crust and spread to coat the crust evenly. Cover the custard with a single layer of sliced bananas and alternate custard and bananas once more.

Chill the pie in the refrigerator for at least 8 hours, until set. Serve chilled.

# CLASSIC APPLE PIE

*Makes* 1 pie

IT SEEMS THAT PEOPLE WHO SHY AWAY FROM PIE MAKING ARE PUT OFF MOSTLY BY THE thought of making the crust. But hopefully now you've mastered the Sweet Pastry Crust (see page 31) and are a true believer. After that, this pie is smooth sailing. Peeling, coring, and slicing the apples can be a bit time consuming, but the more you do it, the easier and quicker it gets. We go to a beautiful orchard every fall for apple picking and then come home and make fresh apple pies. I always freeze, unbaked, at least one assembled pie to use come Thanksgiving, and the rest are gone in an instant. The house smells like a dream.

1 recipe Sweet Pastry Crust, chilled (see page 31)

All-purpose gluten-free flour, for sprinkling (see page 21)

5 firm, tart apples, peeled, cored, and sliced (Granny Smith work well here)

½ cup (100 g) granulated sugar

1 tablespoon (9 g) cornstarch

½ teaspoon pure vanilla extract

½ teaspoon ground cinnamon

½ teaspoon (3 g) kosher salt

GREASE A 9-INCH PIE PLATE AND SET IT ASIDE.

Separate the pastry crust into two disks. Working with one piece at a time, place the dough on a lightly floured piece of unbleached parchment paper. Sprinkle lightly with more flour. Roll out the first piece of dough into an 11-inch round. Roll the round of dough gently onto the rolling pin, and unroll onto the prepared pie plate. Gently press the dough into the pie plate, trim any very rough edges, and tuck the remaining overhung crust under the edges so it sits even with the edge of the pie plate. Place the pie plate in the freezer for 5 minutes to chill. Roll out the other piece of piecrust into an 11-inch round in the same manner. Place the crust, still on the parchment paper, on a flat surface, and transfer to the refrigerator to chill.

Preheat the oven to 375°F. In a large bowl, place the apples, sugar, cornstarch, vanilla, cinnamon, and salt, and stir to coat the apples.

Once chilled, remove the pie plate from the refrigerator. Transfer the apple mixture to the pie shell, piling the apples a bit higher in the center of the pie. Remove the remaining dough from the refrigerator, and invert the dough onto the top of the apples. Carefully remove the remaining sheet of parchment paper. Pinch the top and bottom pie shells together, pinching gently all around the pie plate.

With a very sharp knife, make two ½-inch cuts near the center of the top pie shell to allow steam to escape. Cover the entire pie, both top and bottom, with foil. At this point, the unbaked pie can be frozen and baked at another time.

Place the pie on a rimmed baking sheet and in the middle of the preheated oven, and bake, covered, for 45 minutes. Uncover the top of the pie and bake for another 10 to 15 minutes, until the crust is nicely browned. Allow to cool about 30 minutes, or more, before slicing and serving.

*Shoestring*
SAVINGS | ON A SHOESTRING: $5.83/pie
ON THE SHELF: $13.49/pie

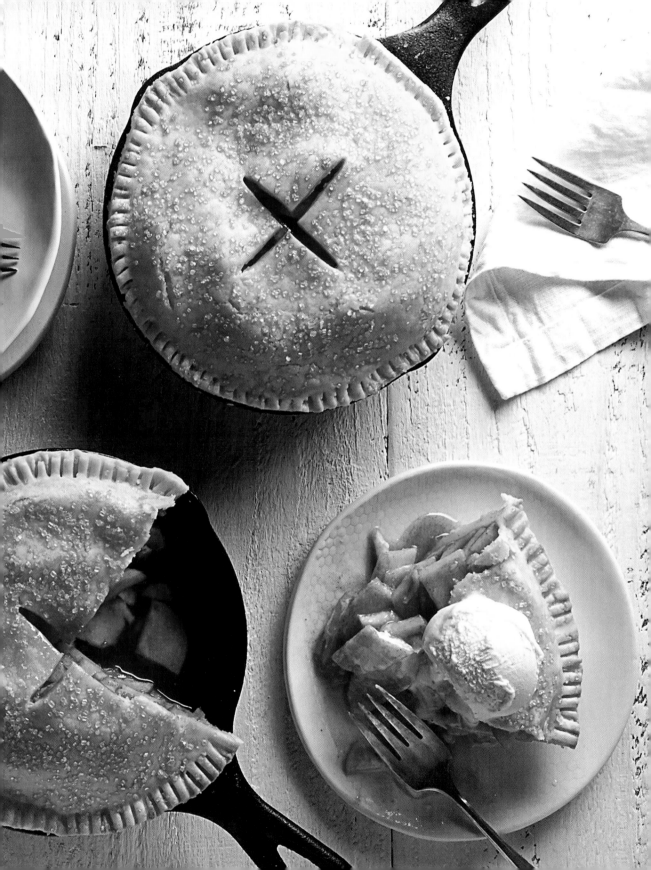

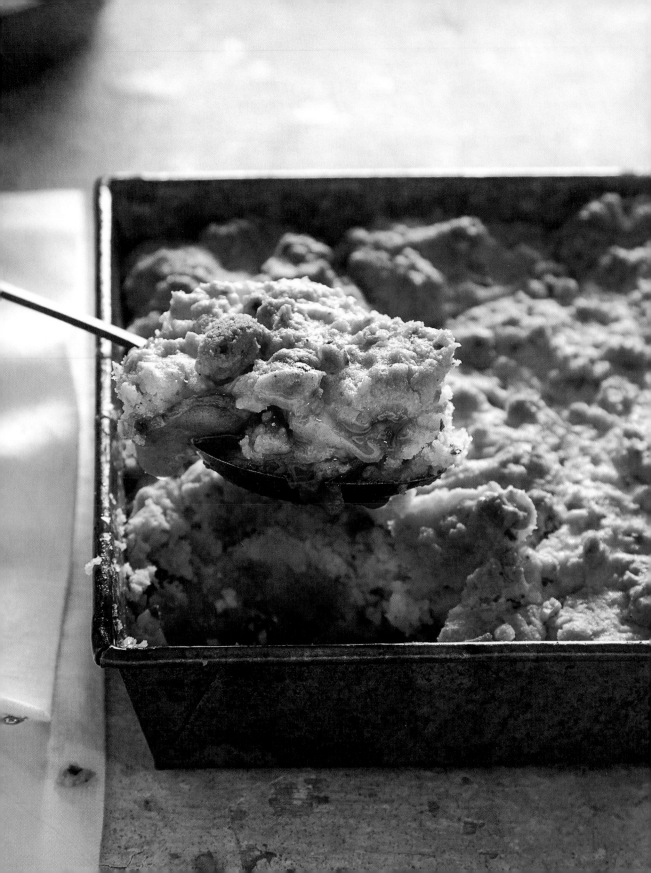

# APPLE CRISP

*Makes* 6 to 8 servings

MAKING THIS APPLE CRISP IS ALMOST AS EASY AS MAKING APPLESAUCE, WHICH ITSELF is a great use of apples that have begun to show signs of age. Once they're peeled, cored, sliced, and cooked down either in a pot on the stovetop or in the oven tucked under an apple crisp, no one minds if the apples were a little bruised or browned. I won't tell.

### FILLING

5 to 6 firm apples, peeled, cored and sliced thinly (Granny Smith work well here)

1 teaspoon ground cinnamon

½ teaspoon (3 g) kosher salt

2 tablespoons (24 g) granulated sugar

### TOPPING

10 tablespoons (140 g) unsalted butter, at room temperature

1 cup (200 g) granulated sugar

1 egg (50 g, weighed out of shell), at room temperature, beaten

2 teaspoons pure vanilla extract

1½ cups (210 g) all-purpose gluten-free flour (see page 21)

½ teaspoon xanthan gum (omit if your blend already contains it)

½ teaspoon (3 g) kosher salt

¼ cup (25 g) certified gluten-free old-fashioned rolled oats

PREHEAT THE OVEN TO 350°F. GREASE A 9-INCH PIE PLATE AND SET IT ASIDE.

To make the filling, in a large bowl, place the apples, cinnamon, salt, and sugar, and stir to combine well. Transfer the filling to the prepared pie plate.

To make the topping, in a large bowl, place the butter and sugar, and beat until light and fluffy. Add the egg and vanilla, and mix to combine well. Add the flour, xanthan gum, salt, and oats, and mix well. The mixture will be thick. Cover the apples with topping, spreading it evenly with wet hands.

Place the pie plate in the center of the preheated oven and bake for about 45 minutes or until the topping is lightly golden brown. Cool at least 20 minutes before slicing and serving.

# CHEESECAKE WITH BUTTER COOKIE CRUST

*Makes* 6 to 8 servings

NOT ONLY IS THE BEAUTIFUL, GOLDEN CRUST AN EXTRA-SPECIAL PART OF THIS RECIPE, the filling is made extra rich with mascarpone cheese and fresh lemon juice and zest. The crust must be blind baked and allowed to cool completely before filling it, steps I encourage you to do a day or so ahead of time, just to make things entirely more pleasant. To prevent the cheesecake from baking unevenly or too quickly, we bake it in a simple water bath. Don't worry—I tell you exactly how to do it.

### CRUST

8 tablespoons (112 g) unsalted butter, at room temperature

¼ cup (50 g) granulated sugar

½ cup (70 g) all-purpose gluten-free flour (see page 21)

¼ teaspoon xanthan gum (omit if your blend already contains it)

½ cup finely ground Butter Cookies (see page 217)

### FILLING

3 (8-ounce) packages cream cheese, at room temperature

8 ounces mascarpone cheese

1½ cups (300 g) granulated sugar

3 eggs (150 g, weighed out of shell), at room temperature, beaten

Juice and finely grated zest of 1 lemon

¼ teaspoon (almost 2 g) kosher salt

PREHEAT THE OVEN TO 350°F. GREASE A 9-INCH PIE PLATE, AND SET IT ASIDE.

To make the crust, in a large bowl, place the butter and the sugar, and beat until light and fluffy. Add the flour, xanthan gum, and ground butter cookies. Mix until all the ingredients are well combined.

Press the mixture into the bottom of the prepared pie plate. Place in the center of the preheated oven, and bake until lightly golden brown, about 20 minutes. Cool completely. In the meantime, make the filling.

In a large bowl, place the cream cheese, and beat until light and fluffy. Add the mascarpone cheese and the sugar, and then the eggs one at a time, mixing after each addition until well blended. Add in the lemon juice and zest, and the salt, and mix to combine.

Pour the filling into the cooled crust and smooth the top. Fill a large ovenproof dish (a 12 × 9-inch roasting pan or other similar dish works well) with water about halfway, and place it on the bottom rack of the preheated oven. Place the cheesecake on the middle rack. Bake for about 1 hour, until the cake is set. If you shake the plate a bit from side to side, the cheesecake should jiggle only slightly in the center.

Turn off the oven and prop the oven door open slightly. Allow the cheesecake to sit in the oven until the temperature drops to about 250°F. Remove from the oven, allow to cool to room temperature. Place the cheesecake in the refrigerator for at least an hour to chill before slicing and serving.

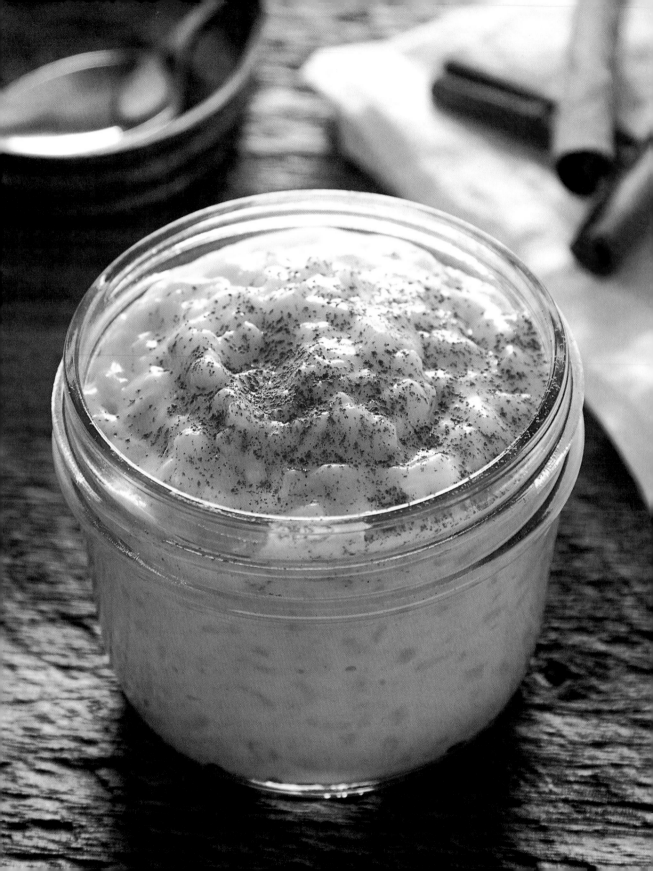

# RICE PUDDING

*Makes* 6 servings

BEFORE I HAD TRIED GOOD, CREAMY RICE PUDDING, IT SOUNDED LIKE MADNESS TO ME. How could rice be dessert? When it's rice pudding, that's how. It's very similar to traditional vanilla pudding, but rice stands in for the cornstarch to make a creamy but substantial pudding.

2 cups (16 fluid ounces) lukewarm water

⅛ teaspoon (almost 1 g) kosher salt

1 tablespoon (14 g) unsalted butter

1 cup short-grain rice (like sushi rice or arborio)

4 cups (32 fluid ounces) milk

½ cup (100 g) granulated sugar

2 teaspoons pure vanilla extract

⅛ teaspoon ground cinnamon

IN A LARGE SAUCEPAN, BRING THE WATER TO A BOIL. ONCE THE WATER IS BOILING, ADD THE salt, butter, and rice, and stir to combine. Reduce the heat to a simmer and cook uncovered for about 10 to 15 minutes or until the rice has absorbed most of the water, leaving behind no more than a bit of thick, starchy water. Be careful not to overcook the rice.

While the rice is cooking, in a separate, medium saucepan, place the milk, sugar, vanilla, and cinnamon, and cook over medium heat until the mixture is simmering. Once the rice in the separate saucepan is cooked, add the simmering milk mixture to the larger saucepan. Cook the rice and milk mixture over medium-low heat, stirring occasionally, until the rice has absorbed most of the milk mixture and the entire mixture has thickened and begins to appear pudding-like, 15 to 20 minutes more. The pudding will thicken as it cools and will set in the refrigerator.

Cool the pudding in the pan for about 15 minutes, then transfer to a large bowl and allow it to cool completely at room temperature. Cover with plastic wrap and refrigerate until set, at least an hour.

# TOPPINGS

# BASIC WHITE FROSTING

*Makes* enough frosting for one 8-inch,
two-layer cake or 24 to 36 cupcakes

THE SALT BALANCES THE SWEETNESS OF THIS FROSTING, WHICH ALLOWS YOU TO USE enough confectioners' sugar to make proper frosting. It has a respectable consistency without being cloyingly sweet.

8 tablespoons (112 g) unsalted butter, at room temperature

8 tablespoons (96 g) nonhydrogenated vegetable shortening

1 teaspoon pure vanilla extract (colorless, if the frosting must be white)

¼ to ½ teaspoon (2 to 3 g) kosher salt

3 to 4 cups (345 to 460 g) confectioners' sugar

2 to 4 tablespoons (1 to 2 fluid ounces) milk

IN THE BOWL OF A STAND MIXER FITTED WITH THE PADDLE ATTACHMENT OR A LARGE BOWL with a handheld mixer, place the butter and shortening, and beat at high speed until light and fluffy. Add the vanilla and ¼ teaspoon of the salt, and beat to combine.

Add 3 cups of the confectioners' sugar, one cup at a time, beating well after each addition. Add the final cup more slowly, beating constantly, until you reach the desired consistency. Add the milk and beat well to smooth out the appearance of the frosting.

Taste a bit of frosting. Add the remaining ¼ teaspoon salt if you wish.

# CITRUS GLAZE

*Makes* enough glaze for 12 standard-size cupcakes

L EMON CUPCAKES (SEE PAGE 224) HAVE EXTRA ZIP WHEN ICED WITH CITRUS GLAZE. The glaze is also delightful drizzled over Pound Cake (see page 236)

1 to 1½ cups (115 to 173 g) confectioners' sugar

2 tablespoons (1 fluid ounce) freshly squeezed lemon juice

IN A MEDIUM-SIZE BOWL, PLACE THE CONFECTIONERS' SUGAR AND THE LEMON JUICE, AND MIX until smooth, adjusting the amount of confectioners' sugar to achieve a thick but pourable glaze. If you find that you have added too much sugar, just add a few drops of water to thin the glaze.

When using the glaze, place whatever cakes you are glazing on a wire rack, pour the glaze evenly over the top, and allow it to set. Chill glazed cakes in the refrigerator to set if your environment is humid.

# SOUR CREAM CHOCOLATE FROSTING

*Makes* enough frosting for one 8-inch, two-layer cake

Making my own dressings, frostings, and sauces is something I started doing many years ago. The ingredients that are essential to these staples not only have long shelf lives but also are already part of an otherwise well-stocked pantry. And, of course, making them yourself means that you can modify the recipes to suit your personal tastes and make only what you need. Good taste at a good price, with no waste.

1 cup (6 ounces) semisweet chocolate chips

4 tablespoons (56 g) unsalted butter

½ cup (113 g) sour cream, at room temperature

1 teaspoon pure vanilla extract

¼ teaspoon (almost 2 g) kosher salt

1½ to 2 cups (173 to 230 g) confectioners' sugar

In a large, microwave-safe bowl, place the chocolate chips and butter. Microwave for 30 seconds at a time, stirring well after each 30-second cycle, until smooth and shiny.

Add the sour cream, vanilla, and salt to the chocolate mixture, and mix by hand until smooth. Gradually add the confectioners' sugar, blending well, until spreadable.

# ROYAL ICING

*Makes* about 1 cup icing

ROYAL ICING BEGINS TO HARDEN UPON EXPOSURE TO THE AIR, SO IT SHOULD BE USED immediately or placed in an airtight container until you are ready to use it. If you store the icing before using it, you will need to add a few drops of water and beat the icing again until it returns to the proper consistency for piping. Once you have used the icing as you have planned, whatever has been iced should be allowed to dry completely at room temperature, which will take several hours, before storing. Royal icing is very useful for decorating cookies at the holidays. Put it in a piping bag with a #2 tip, or just snip off the very corner of a zip-top bag and use it to pipe thin lines of icing in whatever shape you like. I consider it essential for making even the simplest of gingerbread men look authentic (see page 201).

1 cup (115 g) confectioners' sugar

2¼ teaspoons meringue powder

1 tablespoon (½ fluid ounce) lukewarm water, plus more by the ¼ teaspoonful if necessary

Gel food coloring (optional)

IN THE BOWL OF A STAND MIXER FITTED WITH THE PADDLE ATTACHMENT OR A LARGE BOWL with a hand mixer, beat the sugar, meringue powder, and 1 tablespoon of water on low speed until a paste forms. Add a few more drops of water, and raise the mixer speed to medium high. Beat until the mixture thickens enough that the beater leaves a visible trail in the icing. Add more water by the ¼ teaspoonful or less if the icing seems too thick, and more sugar by the teaspoonful if it seems too runny.

Add optional gel food coloring sparingly, blending well after each addition, until the desired color is reached.

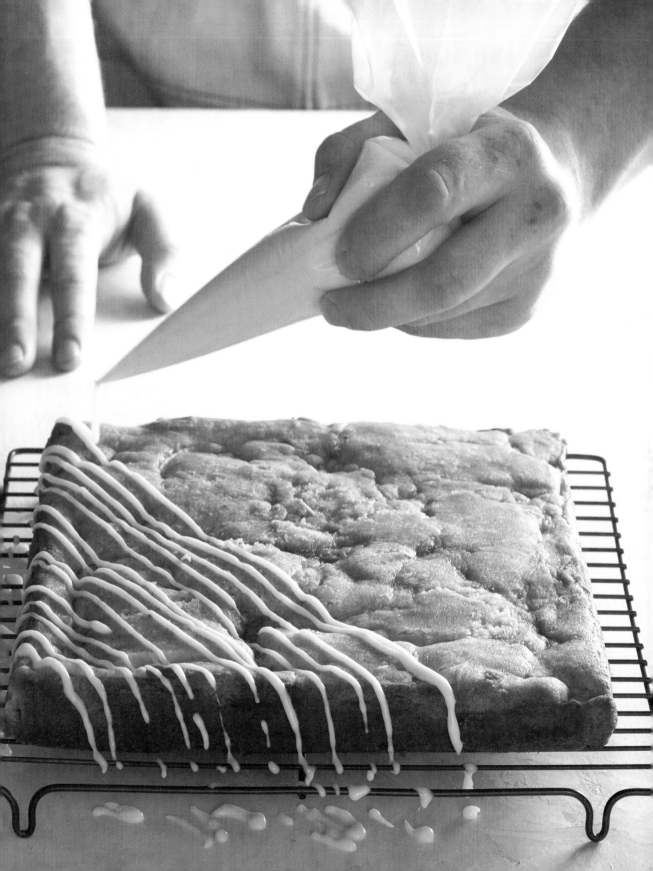

# METRIC CONVERSIONS

The recipes in this book have not been tested with metric measurements, so some variations might occur. Remember that the weight of dry ingredients varies according to the volume or density factor: 1 cup of flour weighs far less than 1 cup of sugar, and 1 tablespoon doesn't necessarily hold 3 teaspoons.

## GENERAL FORMULA FOR METRIC CONVERSION

| | |
|---|---|
| Ounces to grams | multiply ounces by 28.35 |
| Grams to ounces | multiply grams by 0.035 |
| Pounds to grams | multiply pounds by 453.5 |
| Pounds to kilograms | multiply pounds by 0.45 |
| Cups to liters | multiply cups by 0.24 |
| Fahrenheit to Celsius | subtract 32 from Fahrenheit temperature, multiply by 5, divide by 9 |
| Celsius to Fahrenheit | multiply Celsius temperature by 9, divide by 5, add 32 |

## VOLUME (LIQUID) MEASUREMENTS

| | | |
|---|---|---|
| 1 teaspoon | = 1/6 fluid ounce | = 5 milliliters |
| 1 tablespoon | = 1/2 fluid ounce | = 15 milliliters |
| 2 tablespoons | = 1 fluid ounce | = 30 milliliters |
| 1/4 cup | = 2 fluid ounces | = 60 milliliters |
| 1/3 cup | = 2 2/3 fluid ounces | = 79 milliliters |
| 1/2 cup | = 4 fluid ounces | = 118 milliliters |
| 1 cup or 1/2 pint | = 8 fluid ounces | = 250 milliliters |
| 2 cups or 1 pint | = 16 fluid ounces | = 500 milliliters |
| 4 cups or 1 quart | = 32 fluid ounces | = 1,000 milliliters |
| 1 gallon | = 4 liters | |

## WEIGHT (MASS) MEASUREMENTS

| | | |
|---|---|---|
| 1 ounce | = 30 grams | |
| 2 ounces | = 55 grams | |
| 3 ounces | = 85 grams | |
| 4 ounces | = 1/4 pound | = 125 grams |
| 8 ounces | = 1/2 pound | = 240 grams |
| 12 ounces | = 3/4 pound | = 375 grams |
| 16 ounces | = 1 pound | = 454 grams |

## OVEN TEMPERATURE EQUIVALENTS, FAHRENHEIT (F) AND CELSIUS (C)

| | |
|---|---|
| 100°F | = 38°C |
| 200°F | = 95°C |
| 250°F | = 120°C |
| 300°F | = 150°C |
| 350°F | = 180°C |
| 400°F | = 205°C |
| 450°F | = 230°C |

## VOLUME (DRY) MEASUREMENTS

| | |
|---|---|
| 1/4 teaspoon | = 1 milliliter |
| 1/2 teaspoon | = 2 milliliters |
| 3/4 teaspoon | = 4 milliliters |
| 1 teaspoon | = 5 milliliters |
| 1 tablespoon | = 15 milliliters |
| 1/4 cup | = 59 milliliters |
| 1/3 cup | = 79 milliliters |
| 1/2 cup | = 118 milliliters |
| 2/3 cup | = 158 milliliters |
| 3/4 cup | = 177 milliliters |
| 1 cup | = 225 milliliters |
| 4 cups or 1 quart | = 1 liter |
| 1/2 gallon | = 2 liters |
| 1 gallon | = 4 liters |

## LINEAR MEASUREMENTS

| | |
|---|---|
| 1/2 inch | = 1 1/2 cm |
| 1 inch | = 2 1/2 cm |
| 6 inches | = 15 cm |
| 8 inches | = 20 cm |
| 10 inches | = 25 cm |
| 12 inches | = 30 cm |
| 20 inches | = 50 cm |

# ACKNOWLEDGMENTS

To my family, for reasons that are now more than familiar, thank you.

To my editor, Renée Sedliar, I cherish your thoughtfulness, your savvy, your intelligence—and your politics. Where you lead, I will follow.

To my agent, Brandi Bowles, you're my touchstone for each project, from start to finish. I'm grateful, as always, to have you on my side.

To Jean Schwarzwalder, you somehow managed to take this, the book that started it all in 2011, and tell the whole story through photographs that capture where I've been—and where I'm going. You did a masterful job.

To Derek Laughren, I'm not sure what I love more, your skill as a chef and food stylist or your easygoing manner. And thank you for bringing Jesse Breneman onto the team. Not only did he whip heavy cream into beautiful peaks by hand, but he endured our merciless teasing as he toiled.

To everyone else at Da Capo who brought this cookbook to life, including, of course, Amber Morris and Alex Camlin, thank you as always. It was such a pleasure to have you at the photo shoot, Alex. Thank you for coming all that way and for making the cover this book was always meant to have, at last.

And finally, to my blog readers. Whether you've purchased this revised edition to go alongside the first, or whether this is your first introduction to the Shoestring series, I am in your debt. Without you, quite literally none of this is possible. You've changed my life, one recipe at a time!

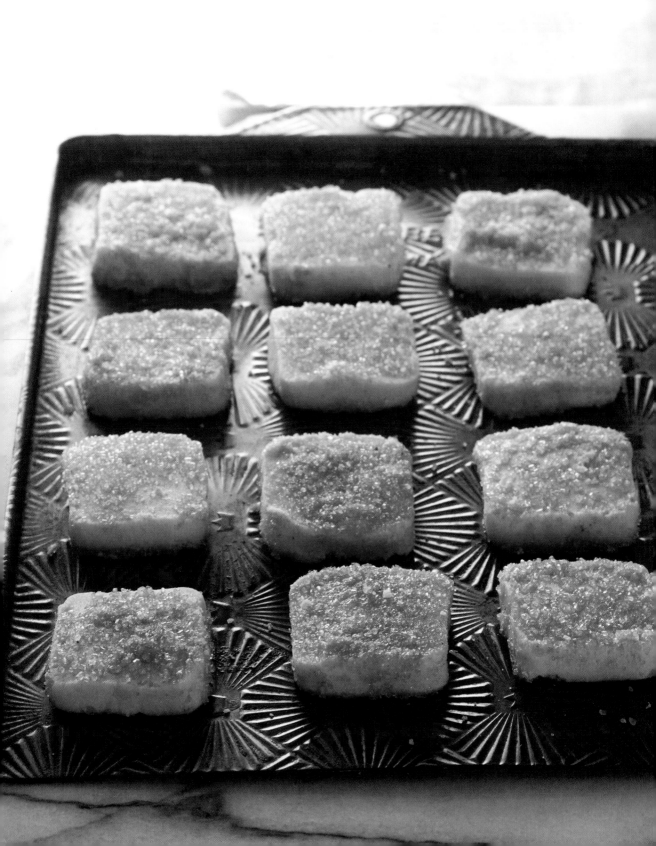

# INDEX

NOTE: Page references in italics indicate photographs.

## A

All-purpose gluten-free flour blends, 19–20
Almonds
    Homemade Crunchy Granola, *74,* 75
Amazon.com, for gluten-free shopping, 15–16
Apple(s)
    Cake, 240, *241*
    Cinnamon Toaster Pastries, 72–73
    Crisp, *252, 253*
    Leek-Sausage Cornbread Stuffing Dinner, 166–67
    making applesauce with, 6

Pie, Classic, 249–50, *251*
    storing, 7
Arepas, *148,* 149
Asian Pork Loin, 180
Asian-style spider strainer, 17

## B

Bagels, Plain, 76–77
Baked Eggplant Parmesan, *134,* 135
Baking ingredients, 11–12
Baking sheets, rimmed, 17
Balloon whisk, 18
Banana(s)
    buying, tip for, 14
    Cream Pie with Graham Cracker Crust, *246, 247–48*
    Muffins, *84,* 85
    overripe, freezing, 6

Pancake Muffins, 68, *69*
Barbecue Sauce, 47
Bar cookies
    Chocolate Chip Brownies, 227
    Flourless Brownies, *228,* 229
    Pumpkin Chocolate Chip Squares, 244
Basic Gum-Free Gluten-Free Flour, 21
Basic White Frosting, 259
Beans
    Black, Scratch, 28
    Chicken Enchiladas, 193
    pantry staples, 11
    Traditional Hummus, 54
Beef
    Meatlove, 168, *169*
    Potpie, 186
    Pot Roast, 192
    Potstickers, *174,* 175

*Beef (cont.)*

    Shepherd's Pie, *184,* 185

    Szechuan Meatballs, 172,
       *173*

Beets, Sweet and Sour, 132

Berry(ies)

    Blueberry Muffins, 82,
       *83*

    Homemade Crunchy
       Granola, *74,* 75

    in season, buying, 14

    Scones, *80,* 81

Better Batter All-Purpose
    Gluten-Free Flour,
    Mock, 21

Better Batter Gluten Free
    Flour, 15, 19–20

Better than Cup4Cup All-
    Purpose Gluten-Free
    Flour, 21

Biscotti, Chocolate Chip,
    212, *213*

Biscuits

    and Sausage Gravy, 91

    Buttermilk, 104–5, *105*

    Drop, *102,* 103

    Sweet Potato, *106,* 107–8

Black and White Cookies,
    214–15

Blender, immersion, 17

Blintzes, Cheese, 89–90

Blueberry(ies)

    Berry Scones, *80,* 81

    Muffins, 82, *83*

Bread Flour, Gluten-Free

    buying whey protein
       isolate for, 20

    homemade blend, 21

Bread(s)

    Brioche, 114, *115*

    Buttermilk Biscuits,
       104–5, *105*

    Cinnamon Rolls, 78–79

    Cornmeal Flatbread, 98

    Crêpes, 126, *127*

    Dinner Rolls, 99–100,
       *101*

    Drop Biscuits, *102,* 103

    English Muffin, *112,* 113

    Flour Tortillas, 121–22, *123*

    Irish Soda, 116–17, *117*

    Old-Fashioned
       Cornbread, *96,* 97

    Plain Bagels, 76–77

    Popovers, *124,* 125

    Pudding, 88

    Pumpkin, *242,* 243

    Soft Pretzels, *118,* 119–20

    stale, uses for, 6

    Sweet Potato Biscuits,
       *106,* 107–8

    White Sandwich, 109–10,
       *111*

Breakfast and brunch

    Apple-Cinnamon Toaster
       Pastries, 72–73

    Banana Muffins, *84,* 85

    Banana Pancake Muffins,
       68, *69*

    Berry Scones, *80,* 81

    Biscuits and Sausage
       Gravy, 91

    Blueberry Muffins, 82, *83*

    Bread Pudding, 88

    Buttermilk Pancakes, *66, 67*

    Cheese Blintzes, 89–90

    Cinnamon Rolls, 78–79

    Coffee Cake, 86–87, *87*

    Easy Oatmeal Breakfast
       Cookies, 71

    Homemade Crunchy
       Granola, *74,* 75

    Oven Hash Brown
       Quiche, *62,* 63

    Plain Bagels, 76–77

    Ricotta Pancakes, *64, 65*

    Soft and Fluffy Waffles,
       70

    Tortilla Española, 60–61

Brioche Bread, 114, *115*

Broccoli

    Cheddar Soup, 161

    Oven Hash Brown
       Quiche, *62,* 63

Brownies

    Chocolate Chip, 227

    Flourless, *228,* 229

Brown rice flour

    Better than Cup4Cup All-
       Purpose Gluten-Free
       Flour, 21

    Mock Better Batter All-
       Purpose Gluten-Free
       Flour, 21

Butter

    buying on sale, 7

    Cookie Crust, Cheesecake
       with, 254–55

    Cookies, *216,* 217–18

    dairy-free, buying, 19

    freezing, 7

Buttermilk

    Biscuits, 104–5, *105*

    Pancakes, *66, 67*

## C

Cakes
    Apple, 240, *241*
    Chocolate Birthday,
        Perfect, *238,* 239
    Chocolate Chip Blondie
        Cupcakes, 226
    Coffee, 86–87, *87*
    Devil's Food, 235
    Lemon Cupcakes, 224,
        *225*
    Pound, 236, *237*
    Yellow, Perfect, 232–34,
        *233*
Carrots
    Glazed, 133
    Shepherd's Pie, *184,* 185
    Sweet and Sour Chicken,
        176, *177*
Carving knife, 17
Cast-iron Dutch oven, 17
Cheddar Broccoli Soup, 161
Cheese
    and Spinach Ravioli,
        142–43
    Arepas, *148,* 149
    Baked Eggplant
        Parmesan, *134,* 135
    Beef Potpie, 186
    Blintzes, 89–90
    buying, 7, 13
    Cheddar Broccoli Soup,
        161
    Cheesecake with Butter
        Cookie Crust, 254–55
    Chicken Enchiladas, 193
    Chicken en Croute, 187

    Crackers, *56,* 57
    dairy-free, buying, 18–19
    Macaroni and, *164,* 165
    Meatlove, 168, *169*
    No-Bake Cheesecake,
        230–31, *231*
    Noodle Kugel, 159
    Oven Hash Brown
        Quiche, *62,* 63
    Polenta Pizza, *156,* 157
    Puffs (Gougères), 43
    Ricotta Gnocchi, 139–40
    Ricotta Pancakes, 64, *65*
    Spinach Dip, 53
    Spinach Pie, 146–47, *147*
    Tomato Polenta, 154, *155*
    Zucchini Pizza, 158
    Zucchini-Stuffed Chicken
        Parmesan Bundles,
        194–95, *195*
Cheesecakes
    No-Bake, 230–31, *231*
    with Butter Cookie Crust,
        254–55
Chef's knife, 17
Chewy Sugar Cookies, 221
Chicken
    and Dumplings Soup,
        188, *189*
    Cream of, Soup, 50
    Enchiladas, 193
    en Croute, 187
    Lemon, Chinese-Style,
        *178,* 179
    Parmesan Bundles,
        Zucchini-Stuffed,
        194–95, *195*
    Potpie, 181–82, *183*

    Stock, 26, *27*
    Sweet and Sour, 176, *177*
    Tortilla Soup, 191
Chinese-Style Hot Sauce, 46
Chocolate
    Birthday Cake, Perfect,
        *238, 239*
    Black and White Cookies,
        214–15
    Chip Biscotti, 212, *213*
    Chip Blondie Cupcakes,
        226
    Chip Brownies, 227
    Chip Cookies, Thick and
        Chewy, *198,* 199
    Chip Pumpkin Squares,
        244
    Cookie Breakup, 219
    Devil's Food Cake, 235
    Easy Oatmeal Breakfast
        Cookies, 71
    Flourless Brownies, *228,*
        229
    Frosting, Sour Cream, 261
    Sandwich Cookies, 220
    Wafer Cookies, Crispy,
        208, *209*
Cinnamon Rolls, 78–79
Citrus Glaze, 260
Classic Apple Pie, 249–50,
    *251*
Coffee Cake, 86–87, *87*
Company website coupons,
    3–4
Condiments, 11
Cookies
    Black and White, 214–15
    Butter, *216,* 217–18

Cookies *(cont.)*

Chocolate Chip, Thick and Chewy, *198,* 199

Chocolate Chip Biscotti, 212, *213*

Chocolate Sandwich, 220

Chocolate Wafer, Crispy, 208, *209*

Cookie Breakup, 219

Ginger, Soft, 202

Gingerbread Men, Crispy, 200, *201*

Graham Crackers, 222–23

Ladyfingers, *210,* 211

Oatmeal Breakfast, Easy, 71

Sugar, Chewy, 221

Sugar, Drop, *206,* 207

Sugar, Soft Frosted, 203–4, *205*

Corn and Zucchini Fritters, 130, *131*

Cornbread

Apple-Leek-Sausage, Stuffing Dinner, 166–67

Old-Fashioned, *96,* 97

Cornmeal

Arepas, *148,* 149

Flatbread, 98

Old-Fashioned Cornbread, *96,* 97

Polenta Pizza, *156,* 157

Spoonbread, *152,* 153

Tomato Polenta, 154, *155*

Cornstarch

Better than Cup4Cup

All-Purpose Gluten-Free Flour, 21

Coupons, shopping with, 2–4

Crackers

Cheese, *56,* 57

Graham, 222–23

Cranberries

Berry Scones, *80,* 81

Homemade Crunchy Granola, *74,* 75

Cream of Chicken Soup, 50

Cream of Mushroom Soup, 49

Cream of Potato Soup, 51

Cream Puffs (Profiteroles), 43

Crêpes, 126, *127*

Crisp, Apple, *252,* 253

Crispy Asian-Style Tofu, 150, *151*

Crispy Chocolate Wafer Cookies, 208, *209*

Crispy Gingerbread Men Cookies, 200, *201*

Cup4Cup All-Purpose Gluten-Free Flour, Better Than, 21

Cup4Cup flours, buying, 19–20

Cupcakes

Chocolate Birthday Cake, 239

Chocolate Chip Blondie, 226

Devil's Food Cake, 235

Lemon, 224, *225*

Vanilla, 232

Cutting boards, 17

**D**

Dairy-free substitutions, 18–19

Dairy products, buying, 13, 14

Desserts

Apple Cake, 240, *241*

Apple Crisp, *252,* 253

Banana Cream Pie with Graham Cracker Crust, *246,* 247–48

Black and White Cookies, 214–15

Butter Cookies, *216,* 217–18

Cheesecake with Butter Cookie Crust, 254–55

Chewy Sugar Cookies, 221

Chocolate Chip Biscotti, 212, *213*

Chocolate Chip Blondie Cupcakes, 226

Chocolate Chip Brownies, 227

Chocolate Sandwich Cookies, 220

Classic Apple Pie, 249–50, *251*

Cookie Breakup, 219

Crispy Chocolate Wafer Cookies, 208, *209*

Crispy Gingerbread Men Cookies, 200, *201*

Devil's Food Cake, 235

Drop Sugar Cookies, *206,* 207

Flourless Brownies, *228,* 229

Graham Crackers, 222–23

Ladyfingers, *210,* 211

Lemon Cupcakes, 224, *225*

No-Bake Cheesecake, 230–31, *231*

Perfect Chocolate Birthday Cake, *238,* 239

Perfect Yellow Cake, 232–34, *233*

Pound Cake, 236, *237*

Profiteroles (Cream Puffs), 43

Pumpkin Bread, *242,* 243

Pumpkin Chocolate Chip Squares, 244

Pumpkin Pie with Ginger Cookie Crust, 245

Rice Pudding, *256,* 257

Soft Frosted Sugar Cookies, 203–4, *205*

Soft Ginger Cookies, 202

Thick and Chewy Chocolate Chip Cookies, *198,* 199

Devil's Food Cake, 235

Digital kitchen scale, 17

Dinner Rolls, 99–100, *101*

Dinners

Apple-Leek-Sausage Cornbread Stuffing Dinner, 166–67

Asian Pork Loin, 180

Beef Potpie, 186

Beef Potstickers, *174,* 175

Chicken and Dumplings Soup, 188, *189*

Chicken Enchiladas, 193

Chicken en Croute, 187

Chicken Potpie, 181–82, *183*

Lemon Chicken, Chinese-Style, *178,* 179

Lo Mein, *170,* 171

Macaroni and Cheese, *164,* 165

Matzoh Ball Soup, 190

Meatlove, 168, *169*

Pot Roast, 192

Shepherd's Pie, *184,* 185

Sweet and Sour Chicken, 176, *177*

Szechuan Meatballs, 172, *173*

Tortilla Soup, 191

Zucchini-Stuffed Chicken Parmesan Bundles, 194–95, *195*

Dips and snacks

Cheese Crackers, *56,* 57

Homemade Jell-O-Style Gelatin, 55

Spinach Dip, 53

Traditional Hummus, 54

Doughs and crusts

Fresh Pasta Dough, *34,* 35

Pâte à Choux, 40–43, *41*

Pizza Dough, 36–37

Savory Olive Oil Crust, 33

Savory Pastry Crust, 32

Sweet Pastry Crust, *30,* 31

Wonton Wrappers, 38–39

Drop Biscuits, *102,* 103

Drop Sugar Cookies, *206,* 207

Dumplings and Chicken Soup, 188, *189*

Dutch oven, 17

## E

Easy Enchilada Sauce, 45

Easy Homemade Tomato Sauce, 48

Easy Oatmeal Breakfast Cookies, 71

Eggplant Parmesan, Baked, *134,* 135

Eggs

for recipes, 13

Oven Hash Brown Quiche, *62,* 63

storing, 7

Tortilla Española, 60–61, *61*

Enamel cast-iron Dutch oven, 17

Enchiladas, Chicken, 193

Enchilada Sauce, Easy, 45

English Muffin Bread, *112,* 113

Equipment, kitchen, 16–18

Expandex modified tapioca starch

about, 20

Gluten-Free Bread Flour, 21

## F

Flatbread, Cornmeal, 98
Flat whisk, 18
Flourless Brownies, *228,* 229
Flours, Gluten-Free
    Basic Gum-Free, 21
    Better Than Cup4Cup
        All-Purpose, 21
    Bread Flour, 21
    commercial all-purpose
        blends, 19–20
    homemade blends, 20–21
    Mock Better Batter
        All-Purpose, 21
    ordering online, 15
    specialty flours, buying,
        20
    storing, 7
Flour Tortillas, 121–22, *123*
Food processor, 17
Freezing foods, 4–5
Fresh Pasta Dough, *34,* 35
Fritters, Corn and Zucchini,
    130, *131*
Frostings
    Basic White, 259
    Sour Cream Chocolate,
        261
Fruit pectin
    Mock Better Batter
        All-Purpose Gluten-
        Free Flour, 21
Fruits. *See also specific fruits*
    fresh, buying, 12–14
    in season, buying, 14
    pantry items, 12
Frying pans, 17

## G

Gelatin, Homemade Jell-O-
    Style, 55
Ginger
    Cookie Crust, Pumpkin
        Pie with, 245
    Cookies, Soft, 202
    Crispy Gingerbread Men
        Cookies, 200, *201*
Glaze, Citrus, 260
Glazed Carrots, 133
Gluten-free cooking
    strategies
    avoiding contamination
        with gluten-
        containing foods, 18
    buy frozen vegetables, 8
    buying sale items in bulk,
        7
    piggyback your meals,
        5–6
    plant a vegetable garden,
        7–8
    practice once-a-month
        cooking, 4–5
    practice once-a-week
        cooking, 4
    smart food storage, 7
    stretch your food, 6
    using online coupons, 2–4
Gluten-free equipment,
    16–18
Gluten-free pantry, 10–16
    baking staples, 11–12
    beans, pasta, and grains, 11
    best shopping values, 16
    frozen vegetables, 12

    fruits and nuts, 12
    grocery items, 11
    oil, vinegar, and
        condiments, 11
    ordering items online,
        14–16
    seasonings, 12
    weekly ingredient
        shopping list, 12–13
Gnocchi
    Potato, *136,* 137–38
    Ricotta, 139–40
Gougères (Cheese Puffs), 43
Graham Cracker Crust,
    Banana Cream Pie
    with, *246,* 247–48
Graham Crackers, 222–23
Grains
    Arepas, *148,* 149
    Cornmeal Flatbread, 98
    Cornmeal Spoonbread,
        *152,* 153
    Easy Oatmeal Breakfast
        Cookies, 71
    Homemade Crunchy
        Granola, *74,* 75
    Lentil Sloppy Joes, *144,*
        145
    Old-Fashioned
        Cornbread, *96,* 97
    Polenta Pizza, *156,* 157
    Rice Pudding, *256,* 257
    Tomato Polenta, 154, *155*
Granola, Homemade
    Crunchy, *74,* 75
Greens
    Spinach and Cheese
        Ravioli, 142–43

Spinach Dip, 53
Spinach Pie, 146–47, *147*
Grocery shopping lists,
    12–13

**H**

Hash Brown Quiche, Oven,
    *62,* 63
Heavy-bottom saucepan, 17
Hoisin Sauce, 47
Homemade Crunchy
    Granola, *74,* 75
Homemade Jell-O-Style
    Gelatin, 55
Hot Sauce, Chinese-Style,
    46
Hummus, Traditional, 54

**I**

Icing, Royal, 262
Immersion blender, 17
Irish Soda Bread, 116–17, *117*

**J**

Jell-O-Style Gelatin,
    Homemade, 55

**K**

Kitchen equipment, 16–18
Kitchen scale, digital, 17

Knives, 17
Kugel, Noodle, 159

**L**

Ladyfingers, *210,* 211
Large pasta pot, 17
Leek-Apple-Sausage
    Cornbread Stuffing
    Dinner, 166–67
Lemon(s)
    Chicken, Chinese-Style,
        *178,* 179
    Citrus Glaze, 260
    Cupcakes, 224, *225*
Lentil Sloppy Joes, *144,* 145
Lo Mein, *170,* 171

**M**

Macaroni and Cheese, *164,*
    165
Matzoh Ball Soup, 190
Meal ingredients
    Barbecue Sauce, 47
    Chicken Stock, 26, *27*
    Chinese-Style Hot Sauce,
        46
    Cream of Chicken Soup,
        50
    Cream of Mushroom
        Soup, 49
    Cream of Potato Soup, 51
    Easy Enchilada Sauce, 45
    Easy Homemade Tomato
        Sauce, 48

Fresh Pasta Dough, *34,* 35
Gougères (Cheese Puffs),
    43
Hoisin Sauce, 47
Pâte à Choux, 40–43, *41*
Pizza Dough, 36–37
Profiteroles (Cream Puffs),
    43
Savory Olive Oil Crust, 33
Savory Pastry Crust, 32
Scratch Black Beans, 28
Sweet and Sour Sauce, 46
Sweet Pastry Crust, *30,* 31
Wonton Wrappers, 38–39
Measuring spoons and cups, 18
Meat
    Apple-Leek-Sausage
        Cornbread Stuffing
        Dinner, 166–67
    Asian Pork Loin, 180
    Beef Potpie, 186
    Biscuits and Sausage
        Gravy, 91
    buying, 13, 14
    freezing, 14
    Meatlove, 168, *169*
    Pot Roast, 192
    Potstickers, *174,* 175
    Shepherd's Pie, *184,* 185
    Szechuan Meatballs, 172,
        *173*
Meatballs, Szechuan, 172, *173*
Meatless meals and sides
    Arepas, *148,* 149
    Baked Eggplant
        Parmesan, *134,* 135
    Cheddar Broccoli Soup,
        161

*Meatless meals and sides (cont.)*

Corn and Zucchini
Fritters, 130, *131*

Cornmeal Spoonbread,
*152,* 153

Crispy Asian-Style Tofu,
150, *151*

Glazed Carrots, 133

Lentil Sloppy Joes, *144,* 145

Noodle Kugel, 159

Polenta Pizza, *156,* 157

Potato Gnocchi, *136,*
137–38

Ricotta Gnocchi, 139–40

Spinach and Cheese
Ravioli, 142–43

Spinach Pie, 146–47, *147*

Sweet and Sour Beets,
132

Tomato Polenta, 154, *155*

Tomato Soup, 160

Zucchini Pizza, 158

Meatlove, 168, *169*

Menu planning, 5–6

Milks, nondairy, 19

Mixer, stand, 17

Mock Better Batter All-
Purpose Gluten-Free
Flour, 21

Muffins

Banana, *84,* 85

Banana Pancake, 68, *69*

Blueberry, 82, *83*

Mushroom, Cream of, Soup,
49

**N**

No-Bake Cheesecake,
230–31, *231*

Nonfat dry milk

Better than Cup4Cup All-
Purpose Gluten-Free
Flour, 21

Nonstick frying pans, 17

Noodle Kugel, 159

Nuts

Bread Pudding, 88

Homemade Crunchy
Granola, *74,* 75

pantry items, 12

**O**

Oats

Easy Oatmeal Breakfast
Cookies, 71

Homemade Crunchy
Granola, *74,* 75

Oils, 11

Old-Fashioned Cornbread,
*96,* 97

Olive Oil Crust, Savory, 33

Onions, storing, 7

Online coupons, 2–4

Online retailers, 14–16

Oven Hash Brown Quiche,
*62,* 63

Oven thermometer, 17

**P**

Pancakes

Buttermilk, *66, 67*

Ricotta, 64, *65*

Paring knife, 17

Pasta

Beef Potpie, 186

Lo Mein, *170,* 171

Macaroni and Cheese,
*164,* 165

Noodle Kugel, 159

pantry staples, 11

Potato Gnocchi, *136,*
137–38

Ricotta Gnocchi, 139–40

Spinach and Cheese
Ravioli, 142–43

Pasta Dough, Fresh, *34,* 35

Pasta pot, 17

Pastries, Apple-Cinnamon
Toaster, 72–73

Pastry brush, 18

Pastry Crust

Savory, 32

Savory Olive Oil, 33

Sweet, *30,* 31

Pâte à Choux, 40–43, *41*

Pecans

Bread Pudding, 88

Peppers

Sweet and Sour Chicken,
176, *177*

Tortilla Soup, 191

Perfect Chocolate Birthday
Cake, *238,* 239

Perfect Yellow Cake, 232–34,
*233*

Pies
  Apple, Classic, 249–50,
    *251*
  Banana Cream, with
    Graham Cracker
    Crust, *246,* 247–48
  Beef Potpie, 186
  Chicken Potpie, 181–82,
    *183*
  Pumpkin, with Ginger
    Cookie Crust, 245
  Shepherd's, *184,* 185
  Spinach, 146–47, *147*
Pizza
  Polenta, *156, 157*
  Zucchini, 158
Pizza Dough, 36–37
Plain Bagels, 76–77
Polenta
  Pizza, *156, 157*
  Tomato, 154, *155*
Popovers, *124, 125*
Pork
  Apple-Leek-Sausage
    Cornbread Stuffing
    Dinner, 166–67
  Biscuits and Sausage
    Gravy, 91
  Loin, Asian, 180
Potato(es)
  buying on sale, 7
  Cream of, Soup, 51
  Gnocchi, *136, 137–*38
  old, cooking with, 6
  Oven Hash Brown
    Quiche, *62,* 63
  Shepherd's Pie, *184, 185*
  storing, 7

Sweet, Biscuits, *106,*
    107–8
Tortilla Española, 60–61,
    *61*
Potato flour
  Mock Better Batter All-
    Purpose Gluten-Free
    Flour, 21
Potato starch
  Basic Gum-Free Gluten-
    Free Flour, 21
  Better than Cup4Cup All-
    Purpose Gluten-Free
    Flour, 21
  Mock Better Batter All-
    Purpose Gluten-Free
    Flour, 21
Potpies
  Beef, 186
  Chicken, 181–82, *183*
Pot Roast, 192
Pots and pans, 17
Potstickers, Beef, *174,* 175
Poultry
  Chicken and Dumplings
    Soup, 188, *189*
  Chicken Enchiladas, 193
  Chicken en Croute, 187
  Chicken Potpie, 181–82,
    *183*
  Chicken Stock, 26, *27*
  Cream of Chicken Soup,
    50
  Lemon Chicken, Chinese-
    Style, *178,* 179
  Sweet and Sour Chicken,
    176, *177*
  Tortilla Soup, 191

Zucchini-Stuffed Chicken
    Parmesan Bundles,
    194–95, *195*
Pound Cake, 236, *237*
Pretzels, Soft, *118,* 119–20
Profiteroles (Cream Puffs), 43
Puddings
  Bread, 88
  Rice, *256,* 257
Pumpkin
  Bread, *242, 243*
  Chocolate Chip Squares,
    244
  Pie with Ginger Cookie
    Crust, 245

Q

Quiche, Oven Hash Brown,
    *62,* 63

R

Raisins
  Easy Oatmeal Breakfast
    Cookies, 71
  Homemade Crunchy
    Granola, *74, 75*
  Irish Soda Bread, 116–17,
    *117*
  Pumpkin Bread, *242, 243*
Ravioli, Spinach and Cheese,
    142–43
Rice
  Lentil Sloppy Joes, *144,* 145
  Pudding, *256, 257*

Ricotta Gnocchi, 139–40
Ricotta Pancakes, 64, *65*
Rimmed metal baking
    sheets, 17
Rolling pin, 18
Rolls
    Cinnamon, 78–79
    Dinner, 99–100, *101*
Royal Icing, 262

**S**

Sandwich Bread, White,
    109–10, *111*
Santoku knife, 17
Saucepans, 17
Sauces
    Barbecue, 47
    Enchilada, Easy, 45
    Hoisin, 47
    Hot, Chinese-Style, 46
    Sweet and Sour, 46
    Tomato, Easy Homemade,
        48
Sausage
    Apple-Leek Cornbread
        Stuffing Dinner,
        166–67
    Gravy, Biscuits and, 91
Savory Olive Oil Crust, 33
Savory Pastry Crust, 32
Scale, digital, 17
Scones, Berry, *80,* 81
Scratch Black Beans, 28
Seasonings, 12
Serrated carving knife, 17
Shepherd's Pie, *184,* 185

Silicone spatulas, 18
Silicone spoons, 18
Sloppy Joes, Lentil, *144,* 145
Small paring knife, 17
Soft and Fluffy Waffles, 70
Soft Frosted Sugar Cookies,
    203–4, *205*
Soft Ginger Cookies, 202
Soft Pretzels, *118,* 119–20
Soups
    Cheddar Broccoli, 161
    Chicken and Dumplings,
        188, *189*
    Cream of Chicken, 50
    Cream of Mushroom, 49
    Cream of Potato, 51
    Matzoh Ball, 190
    Tomato, 160
    Tortilla, 191
Sour Cream Chocolate
    Frosting, 261
Soy sauce, storing, 7
Spatulas, 18
Specialty gluten-free flour
    blends, 20
Spider strainer, 17
Spinach
    and Cheese Ravioli,
        142–43
    Dip, 53
    Pie, 146–47, *147*
Spoonbread, Cornmeal, *152,*
    153
Spoons, wooden or silicone,
    18
Springform pans, 17
Squash. *See* Pumpkin;
    Zucchini

Stand mixer, 17
Stock, Chicken, 26, *27*
Sugar Cookies
    Chewy, 221
    Drop, *206,* 207
    Soft Frosted, 203–4, *205*
Supermarket websites and
    coupons, 3
Sweet and Sour Beets, 132
Sweet and Sour Chicken,
    176, *177*
Sweet and Sour Sauce, 46
Sweet Pastry Crust, *30,* 31
Sweet Potato Biscuits, *106,*
    107–8
Szechuan Meatballs, 172, *173*

**T**

Tamari, storing, 7
Tapioca starch/flour
    Basic Gum-Free Gluten-
        Free Flour, 21
    Better than Cup4Cup All-
        Purpose Gluten-Free
        Flour, 21
    Mock Better Batter All-
        Purpose Gluten-Free
        Flour, 21
Thermometer, oven, 17
Thick and Chewy Chocolate
    Chip Cookies, *198,*
    199
Toaster Pastries, Apple-
    Cinnamon, 72–73
Tofu, Crispy Asian-Style,
    150, *151*

Tomato(es)
  Chinese-Style Hot Sauce,
    46
  Easy Enchilada Sauce, 45
  hothouse, buying, 14
  Polenta, 154, *155*
  Polenta Pizza, *156,* 157
  Pot Roast, 192
  Sauce, Easy Homemade,
    48
  Soup, 160
  Tortilla Soup, 191
Toppings
  Basic White Frosting, 259
  Citrus Glaze, 260
  Royal Icing, 262
  Sour Cream Chocolate
    Frosting, 261
Tortilla Española, 60–61, *61*
Tortillas
  Chicken Enchiladas, 193
  Flour, 121–22, *123*
Tortilla Soup, 191
Traditional Hummus, 54

## V

Vegetable peeler, 18
Vegetables. *See also specific
  vegetables*

Chicken Potpie, 181–82,
  *183*
fresh, buying, 12–14
frozen, buying, 8, 12
growing your own, 7–8
in season, buying, 14
Vinegars, 11

## W

Waffles, Soft and Fluffy, 70
Whey protein isolate
  about, 20
  Gluten-Free Bread Flour,
    21
Whisks, 18
White Frosting, Basic, 259
White rice flour
  Basic Gum-Free Gluten-
    Free Flour, 21
  Better than Cup4Cup All-
    Purpose Gluten-Free
    Flour, 21
  Mock Better Batter All-
    Purpose Gluten-Free
    Flour, 21
White Sandwich Bread,
  109–10, *111*
Wonton Wrappers, 38–39
Wooden spoons, 18

## X

Xanthan gum
  Better than Cup4Cup All-
    Purpose Gluten-Free
    Flour, 21
  Mock Better Batter All-
    Purpose Gluten-Free
    Flour, 21
  note about, 15

## Z

Zucchini
  and Corn Fritters, 130,
    *131*
  Pizza, 158
  Shepherd's Pie, *184,* 185
  Stuffed Chicken Parmesan
    Bundles, 194–95, *195*

# ABOUT THE AUTHOR

Nicole Hunn is the personality behind the popular *Gluten-Free on a Shoestring* blog and book series. She has been featured in high-profile national print and broadcast outlets, including the *New York Times*, *Parade* magazine, *Better Homes and Gardens*, *Parents* magazine, Epicurious.com, ABC News, *The Better Show*, and many others.

Nicole has also been a contributing gluten-free expert for SheKnows.com Food and *Living Without* and *Gluten-Free Living* magazines. She lives in Westchester County, New York, with her husband and three children. For more information and recipes, please visit www.glutenfreeonashoestring.com.

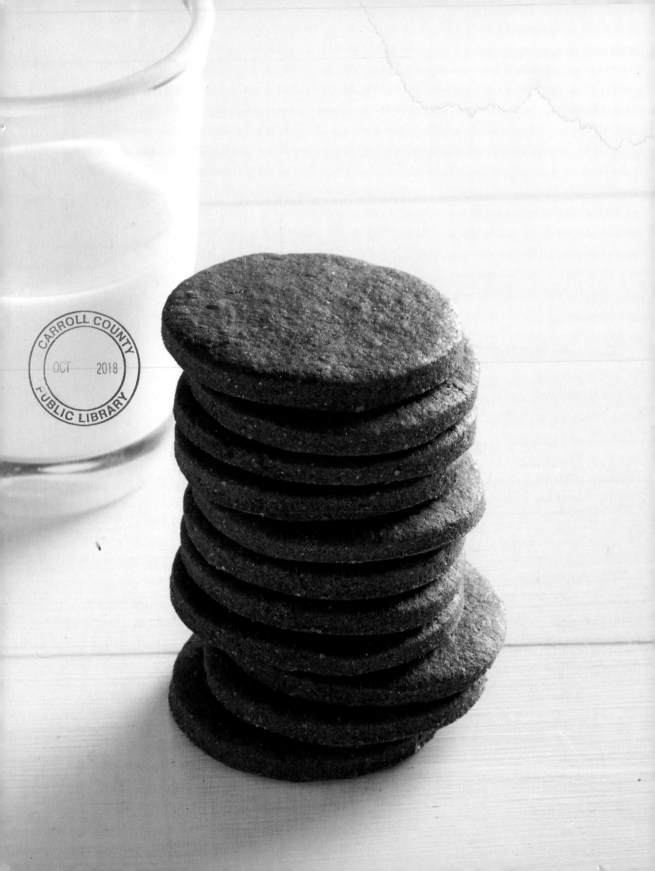
CARROLL COUNTY
OCT 2018
PUBLIC LIBRARY